HANDBOOK OF CONTRACEPTION AND SEXUAL HEALTH

Offering a comprehensive guide to contraception and sexual health, the new edition of this practical handbook has been fully updated. It takes an integrated approach to sexual health and now includes additional content on sexually transmitted infections as well as assessment skills.

Giving clear and detailed information about all contraceptive methods, including how to use them, contra-indications, interactions and common patient anxieties, the *Handbook of Contraception and Sexual Health* is an essential read for all nurses, midwives and allied health professionals working in community heath and primary care settings.

- All chapters have been fully updated with the latest research and methods.
- There are additional chapters on the consultation process, progestogen pills and STIs, and a newly written anatomy and physiology chapter.
- Each chapter takes into account relevant UKMEC guidelines and includes self-assessment exercises.

Suzanne Everett is Senior Lecturer and Module Leader for the Reproductive Sexual Health Module at Middlesex University, UK, and a Senior Nurse Practitioner at Camberwell Sexual Health Clinic, Kings College NHS Hospital, UK.

D0217434

HANDBOOK OF CONTRACEPTION AND SEXUAL HEALTH

THIRD EDITION

SUZANNE EVERETT

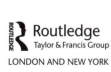
Routledge
Taylor & Francis Group
LONDON AND NEW YORK

First edition published 1998
by Baillière Tindall

Second edition published 2004
by Baillière Tindall

This edition published 2014
by Routledge
2 Park Square, Milton Park, Abingdon, Oxon, OX14 4RN

and by Routledge
711 Third Avenue, New York, NY 10017

Routledge is an imprint of the Taylor & Francis Group, an informa business

British Library Cataloguing in Publication Data
A catalogue record for this book is available from the British Library

Library of Congress Cataloging-in-Publication Data
Everett, Suzanne, author.
[Handbook of contraception and reproductive sexual health]
Handbook of contraception and sexual health / Suzanne Everett. —
Third edition.
p. ; cm.
Preceded by Handbook of contraception and reproductive sexual health /
Suzanne Everett. 2nd ed. 2014.
I. Title.
RG136
618.1'8—dc23   2013026286

ISBN: 978-0-415-65988-8 (hbk)
ISBN: 978-0-415-65989-5 (pbk)
ISBN: 978-0-203-07459-6 (ebk)

Typeset in Sabon by
Keystroke, Station Road, Codsall, Wolverhampton

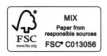

Printed and bound in Great Britain by
TJ International Ltd, Padstow, Cornwall

Dedicated to Mike Skelton, Jon and Isobel Everett

CONTENTS

ILLUSTRATIONS

FIGURES

TABLES

ACKNOWLEDGEMENTS

No book is ever written by one person, without the help and support of other people. I would very much like to thank colleagues who I work with or have worked with in sexual health for their encouragement.

Finally, without the support of Jon, Isobel and my family it would not have been possible to complete this third edition.

THE CONSULTATION

- Introduction
- The consultation
- History taking
- Sexual history taking
- The client
- The nurse–client relationship
- Confidentiality and ethics
- Clinical guidance
- Off-label prescribing
- Quick starting
- Bridging

INTRODUCTION

This book aims to offer a comprehensive introduction to the role of the nurse working in contraception. It addresses some of the problems encountered during consultations, and offers the opportunity to test and evaluate your knowledge through self-assessment questions. The answers to these questions are discussed at the end of each chapter.

Family planning is now usually referred to as reproductive sexual health and, as a profession, it is constantly changing as new methods of contraception become available and new research is published. All health professionals are accountable for their own actions, and as management procedures may vary in hospital trusts and GP practices, it is important that you regularly update and understand policies within your workplace, which may be different from this book. It is vital for professionals to keep their knowledge updated. There are several ways to ensure that this happens:

- By becoming an associate member of the Faculty of Sexual and Reproductive Healthcare, which provides clinical guidance on practice within sexual health, journals and conferences.
- By undertaking psychosexual seminar work which involves reflecting on the nurse–client relationship. By looking at the feelings evoked in the nurse–client relationship in this way, problems encountered are seen from a new perspective, helping the nurse's approach to them in the future.
- By keeping a reflective diary (Benner, 1994), insight can be gained through reflecting and thinking about clinical encounters, which can improve future clinical practice.

THE CONSULTATION

During a consultation you are in a unique position to give men and women the opportunity to talk about intimate areas of their sexual life and anxieties they may have. However, this will only happen when clients feel they are free to discuss any anxiety or problem. Sometimes clients will give you clues to a problem as they are about to leave the room. Sometimes we miss these clues because we are in a rush or fail to recognize the significance of the clue and only realize its meaning on reflection. In some situations we may neglect a statement because we have become caught up in our own agenda. Clients may reveal information about themselves which may be upsetting and shocking to you; if your body language, tone of voice or expression shows this then they will feel that they are unable to disclose any further information for fear of being reproached and judged. It is important never to assume that all clients are heterosexual: reproductive sexual health is not just about preventing pregnancy, but about disease prevention, health promotion and education.

During a consultation, ensure that you are free of interruptions and that total privacy is maintained. Give clients the opportunity to ask questions. Try and ask open-ended questions, for example, 'Do you ever have pain or any difficulties during sexual intercourse?' rather than a closed question such as 'You don't have any pain during intercourse?' which only offers the client the opportunity to say 'no'. Open-ended questions give clients room to bring up problems associated with the area of questioning. Open-ended questions can allow clients to express problems which may in fact be commonplace; sometimes clients can feel that they are the only one having difficulties with, for example, a method of contraception, and knowing that they are not alone can be reassuring.

When undertaking any procedure involving a client, it is important to obtain their consent. For a client to give informed consent you should explain carefully why this procedure is necessary and what it involves. When performing intimate examinations such as vaginal or testicular examinations, you should maintain the client's privacy, allowing them to feel safe without fear of being interrupted by your colleagues or viewed from windows by strangers. Discuss with your client whether they would like a chaperone for any intimate examination.

If you give clients freedom to talk in a non-judgemental environment, then even if they choose not to disclose a problem at an initial consultation, they may return in the future knowing they can feel safe to talk freely.

It is always a good idea to speak to your clients on their own; this ensures that you are gaining their consent and that they are not being coerced into a decision. Young people are usually seen on a one-to-one basis and this is incorporated into the consultation. This is to ensure that they are not being groomed or pressurized into sexual intercourse, and that you are giving the best possible care with all the information available. Increasingly, all consultations are on a one-to-one basis and this should be promoted, as clients do not always divulge full information about their sexual histories in front of sexual partners or relatives. By seeing men and women individually we will ensure that a full history is obtained, and can address issues of sexual abuse and domestic violence. Relatives who interpret for clients may not fully understand the relevance of questions asked and may not translate all questions and answers completely; as a result we may not be able to ensure that full consent has been obtained from them. Following the introduction of the Mental Capacity Act in 2007, it is vital that full consent has been gained. To ensure that this happens, qualified interpreters and signers should be used if needed to make sure the client understands and has the mental capacity to consent.

3

The consultation

CASE STUDY 1.1

A 34-year-old woman attends with her husband for contraception. The husband walks into the consultation room, so you ask him to wait outside. He appears cross and says his wife wants him in the room; you explain that it is your department's policy* to see clients individually, and he relents and leaves the room. When the woman and you are alone, she says that she did not want him in the room, as he does not want her to use contraception and wants her to get pregnant; she does not want to do this at this time. You discuss whether she is being emotionally or physically abused and this does not appear to be the case, and you offer help if this changes. You are then able to discuss why she is unable to express herself fully with her husband, and offer contraception.

Note:
* Not all sexual health departments follow this policy, so it is important to ascertain what is the practice in your area; if there is not a policy in place you may wish to discuss how you all ensure a complete history has been taken.

HISTORY TAKING

At initial consultations with clients, a full medical history should be taken and updated at regular intervals, which must be dated and documented in the notes for future reference. A complete history includes the general health of the client in the past and present, their gynaecological and sexual health, contraceptive history, and the health of their immediate family. Clients can feel threatened by personal questions, especially if they are asked immediately on arrival; try to establish a rapport first by finding out the reason for their attendance. Often, by finding out why a client is attending, other questions that you need to ask will be answered as a by-product. However, you will need to ask questions which should be open-ended, such as 'Do you ever have any premenstrual symptoms?' or 'Do you ever have migraines?' If a client does have a problem you will need to find out more details: for example, if a client has migraines ask her to describe them and their frequency. You will still need to ask specific questions to eliminate contra-indications to different methods of contraception such as 'When you have a migraine do you ever see flashing lights or have loss of vision?' Taking a detailed history can take time but can help nurture a good relationship between you and your clients. It can also create the opportunity for them to discuss issues for which insufficient time was given previously.

SEXUAL HISTORY TAKING

Increasingly, contraceptive and genito-urinary medicine services are combining or offering similar care to streamline services to clients. With the incidence of sexually transmitted infections rising, it is important to discuss sexually transmitted infections with men and women. Many clients believe they will know if they become infected, and do not realize that they may be asymptomatic. In *The Face of Global Sex* report (Durex network, 2010) the Durex network looked at 15 European countries giving a KAP score to represent young people's knowledge, attitudes and practices. It was found that for every year in delay in starting sexual health education there was a drop in KAP score. This corroborates with earlier *Face of Global Sex* work which shows that having increasing numbers of sexual partners is linked to adverse sexual health. This research highlights how little young people know about sexual health and how important it is to promote safe sex practices. We should always try to encourage women and their partners to go for screening once they commence a new sexual relationship, and also when they have had unprotected sexual intercourse. Increasing knowledge in sexual health was seen in *The Face of Global Sex* report (Durex network, 2010) to correlate with delayed commencement of sexual intercourse, and decreased numbers of sexual partners. As health professionals, we need to be accessible to clients and help empower them with knowledge of sexual health and contraception.

THE CLIENT

Clients who attend for advice on contraception can vary not only in the cultural and religious beliefs they hold, but they may also have very different attitudes and values about relationships and sexuality. The decisions and problems a client will encounter will depend on where they are in their life: for example, an unplanned pregnancy may be a disaster to a client aged either 15 or 50 for very different reasons, and the decision they make about the pregnancy will be from different perspectives.

Clients who are under 16 years of age may have taken some time to gain enough courage to attend a family planning clinic, and as a result may feel embarrassed and awkward. Often younger clients may attend with a friend and there may be anxiety over confidentiality, especially if the client is under the age of 16 (see Confidentiality and ethics, page 5). They may have already commenced sexual intercourse and require emergency contraception or already be pregnant. Research (Smith, 1993) has shown that the teenage pregnancy rate is higher in deprived areas, but the abortion rate is higher in affluent areas. The abortion rate may be higher in affluent areas for a number of reasons such as social and parental pressure, or that girls from these areas may know how to access abortion services and have the support of their parents. They may have career plans and see a future ahead (Simms, 1993), while teenagers living in deprived areas may decide to continue with a pregnancy because of lack of access to abortion services. Alternatively, they may not have career plans and see a pregnancy as their future.

Older clients may feel just as awkward as younger clients but for different reasons. They may not have discussed intimate areas of their sexual life with anyone, and may find the situation embarrassing. Society tends to portray clients over the age of 65 as disinterested in sexual intercourse; however, research shows that this is far from the truth (Steinke, 1994). Nevertheless, with increasing age clients may need to adapt their sexual relationships depending on their health, and may wish to discuss this. Often the impact of chronic diseases and medications on sexuality are not fully discussed with clients and their partners. It may take clients some time before they are able to pluck up the courage to discuss these implications, or are given the opportunity by professionals to discuss them.

THE NURSE–CLIENT RELATIONSHIP

During a consultation a relationship develops between the nurse and the client where feelings and emotions may be expressed. Many clients who consult have no problems and attend for contraceptive advice and supplies; however, other clients may have anxieties and problems that take a great deal of courage to discuss. It is during consultations where there are problems that the recognition of feelings evident within the consultation can help illuminate these problems. This can be sufficient to relieve an anxiety or may bring a hidden problem out into the open, where it can be looked at more closely.

Recognizing the type of emotion expressed in a consultation can be difficult, and sometimes you may only be able to recognize it on reflection once a client has left. Reflection and psychosexual seminar training can help improve and increase your skills in this area. There are several reasons why we may fail to recognize feelings or acknowledge a problem. Sometimes we lack the confidence to discuss intimate areas with clients and need a great deal of courage to pursue an issue, but this does become easier with practice. On other occasions our minds may be fixed on our own agenda, which will stop us listening to the client. For example, there may be a very busy clinic and you may feel pressurized to 'hurry things along' or something the client says may trigger a memory or anxiety in your own personal life. You may have a strong desire 'to make things better for the client'. However, listening and being there for them is actually what they want, and learning to do this can be difficult initially. There may be occasions when you feel you are not establishing a relationship with the client and are unsure why this is so.

There are several ways to improve your skills in your relationship with your client:

- By practising listening and recalling conversations. Careful listening can help us pick up clues about how the client feels. Listening will also give you information about the client, which you will need to refer back to as clients will notice very quickly if you are not listening to what they are talking about.
- By learning to observe the body language of your clients. You can practise this by watching people around you.
- What is the client not saying, what are the feelings you are picking up through her body language, tone of voice, facial expression?
- By undertaking Balint seminar training. This is where a group of nurses meet for a set period of time with a seminar leader to discuss the nurses' work. As a group they listen and focus on the feelings invoked by the work; this helps the nurses to look at their work from a new perspective.
- Finally, a personal reflective diary of your work can help improve your skills.

CONFIDENTIALITY AND ETHICS

All clients have the right to expect that information about themselves or others which is divulged during a consultation will remain confidential. Confidentiality should be respected and only broken in exceptional situations such as if the health, welfare or safety of someone other than the client is at serious risk. If possible, clients should be sensitively encouraged to discuss exceptional areas with people involved themselves. Doctors/nurses who breach confidentiality must be able to show good reason for making this decision (NMC, 2008), which would be an ethical decision. Ethics are the moral code by which a nurse's behaviour is governed within their work with clients and their families and the colleagues with whom they work.

Clients under the age of 16 are often concerned that any disclosures about their sexual life will be divulged to their parents. This may prevent clients from seeking help with contraception, resulting in unprotected sexual intercourse. Following the Gillick case, the House of Lords (BMA *et al.*, 1993) established that people under the age of 16 are able to give consent to medical treatment, regardless of age, if they are able to understand what is proposed and the implications and consequences of the treatment. When clients under the age of 16 consult, doctors or nurses should consider the following issues known as the Fraser guidelines:

■ Whether the client understands the treatment, its implications and the risks and benefits of it.
■ Health care professionals should encourage young clients to discuss their consultation with their parents, and their reasons for not wanting to do this. However, confidentiality will still be respected.
■ Professionals should consider whether clients are likely to have sexual intercourse without contraception. They should also consider whether the mental and physical health of the client would suffer if the client was not to receive contraception. Finally, it is important that the client's best interests are taken into account which may mean giving contraception and advice without parental consent.

Following the Data Protection Act 1984 and Access to Health Records Act 1990, clients have the right to have access to their written and computerized records. Where a client is under the age of 16 they may have access to their records if they are able to show an understanding of the reason for the application (Belfield, 1997). If a parent or guardian wishes to have access to these records this will not be permitted unless the client gives consent. If by giving a client access to their records another person's confidentiality would be breached, then information about the other person should be withheld.

It is useful to think about these areas of confidentiality, as clients (especially young clients) will often be concerned about this area, and you will need to be able to respond to this anxiety sensitively.

CLINICAL GUIDANCE

United Kingdom Medical Eligibility Criteria (FSRH, 2009a)

All health professionals work to guidelines; in sexual health clinicians work to the United Kingdom Medical Eligibility Criteria which are based on the World Health Guidance for Contraception. These guidelines are developed and published by the Faculty of Sexual and Reproductive Healthcare. The United Kingdom Medical Eligibility Criteria (UKMEC) give clear guidance on whether you can prescribe a method of contraception for someone with a medical condition (see Table 1.1).

Table 1.1 UKMEC guidance

UKMEC	Guidance
1	A condition for which there is no restriction for the use of the contraceptive method.
2	A condition where the advantages of using the method generally outweigh the theoretical or proven risks.
3	A condition where the theoretical or proven risks generally outweigh the advantages of using the method. The provision of a method requires expert clinical judgement and/or referral to a specialist contraceptive provider, since use of the method is not usually recommended unless other more appropriate methods are not available or not acceptable.
4	A condition which represents an unacceptable risk if the contraceptive method is used.

Throughout this book the UKMEC criteria will be referred to in order to highlight conditions where certain methods of contraception are not suitable. The full UKMEC guidelines are available from the Faculty of Sexual and Reproductive Healthcare.

OFF-LABEL PRESCRIBING

This is where a medication is licensed but used outside its licence. There are many instances where this practice may be advised, one of which is quick starting contraception. There are many more examples where this happens and prescribers need to be aware of these. Prescribers should be able to justify their practice and this practice should be supported by published evidence for this indication; you should be aware that liability sits with the prescriber, the supplier and the dispenser.

QUICK STARTING

This is a practice where clients commence a method of contraception immediately rather than wait to commence with their next period. Quick starting can offer women contraceptive cover faster with no strong adverse effects. Women should always be offered the choice of commencement; if they wish to commence immediately then pregnancy should be excluded. If pregnancy cannot be excluded you should assess the client for emergency contraception, and discuss with the client what they would do if they became pregnant. Quick starting on progestogen pills, combined pills or the progestogen implant is endorsed by the Faculty of Sexual and Reproductive Healthcare if a women wishes to start immediately and is at continued risk of pregnancy. IUDs, IUS, injectables and Co-cyprindiol are not recommended for quick starting (FSRH, 2010a). Clients should be advised how long they will need to use alternative contraception when quick starting, and the need to perform a pregnancy test in three to four weeks' time to exclude pregnancy.

BRIDGING

If a woman cannot start her chosen method immediately, she can use a bridging method like the combined methods or the progestogen pill until pregnancy has been excluded. A pregnancy test should be performed in three to four weeks' time and, if negative, the chosen method commenced.

Sources of useful information on bridging and quick starting are the Faculty of Sexual and Reproductive Healthcare (www.fsrh.org); the British Association of Sexual Health and HIV gives guidance on STIs (www.bashh.org). If you have a patient who is pregnant or concerned about the effects of medications on pregnancy the UK Teratology Information Service is a helpful resource (www.uktis.org).

ANATOMY AND PHYSIOLOGY

2

- Introduction
- Male reproduction system
- Male hormones
- Production of sperm
- Female reproduction system
- Female hormones
- Sexual intercourse
- The Male
- The Female
- The effect of age on men and women
- Further reading

INTRODUCTION

The male and female reproductive systems are important for procreation; the creation of offspring. They may be used to allow expression of sexual desires and emotional intimacy; they may adversely be used to exert power and inflict violence. Understanding the anatomy and physiology of these systems and the influence of hormones is vital for professionals working in sexual health areas to be able to differentiate between normal and abnormal. For example, understanding the difference between physiological discharge and pathological discharge is a useful tool when educating women on fertility awareness or when discussing vaginal infections such as bacterial vaginosis.

ACTIVITY

You may find it useful to continue your reading after this chapter with Chapter 3, 'Natural family planning methods: fertility awareness'.

MALE REPRODUCTION SYSTEM

The male reproductive system includes the **penis** and two **testes**. The testes are located in the **scrotum**. The scrotum consists of skin and subcutaneous tissue.

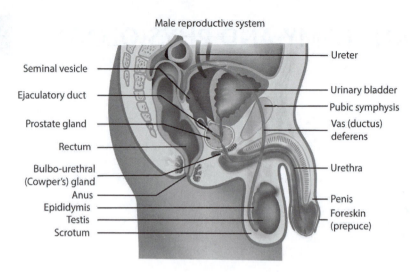

Figure 2.1 Sagital section of the male reproductive organs

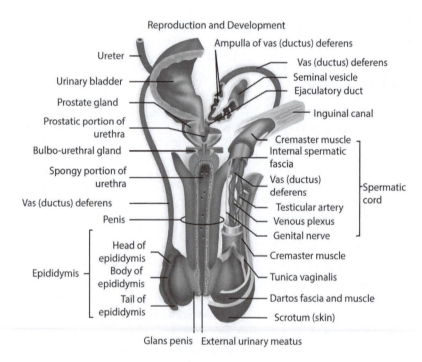

Figure 2.2 Internal male reproductive system

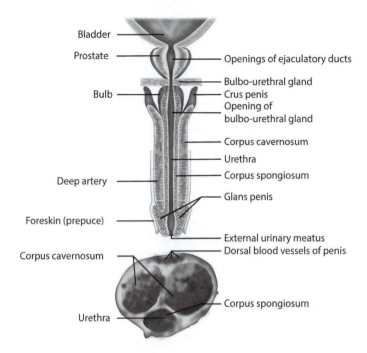

Figure 2.3 Sagital section of the penis

A vertical septum of subcutaneous tissue divides it into two parts, each containing one testis. There are approximately 500 **seminiferous tubules** per testis. The tubules are divided by fibrous septae and surrounded by the **tunica albuginea**. Each tubule is 30 to 70cm long. The location of the testes, outside the abdominal cavity, provides a temperature about 3°C below normal body temperature. This lower temperature is necessary for the production of viable sperm. Interstitial tissue between the seminiferous tubules contains connective tissue, blood vessels, lymphatics and **Leydig cells** which produce **testosterone.** In each testis there are tubules and ducts which form the **epididymis** which then leads on to become the **vas deferens;** this enlarges to become the **ampulla.** The **seminal vesicle** joins each vas deferens at the lower end of the ampulla and these tubes are known as the ejaculatory ducts. The ejaculatory ducts then fuse to the urethra in the **prostate gland** to become one duct: the **prostatic urethra.** The prostatic urethra will then carry semen and urine, and the **bulbo-urethral gland** (Cowper's gland) joins the **urethra** which enters the penis. The penis comprises three cylindrical bodies: two dorsal corpora cavernosa and one corpus spongiosum. The urethra ends at the **external urethral meatus.** The head of the penis is usually covered by the **prepuce** or **foreskin** which can be removed in circumcision.

The seminal vesicles, prostate gland and bulbo-urethral gland are all accessory sex glands which provide sperm with a transport medium and nutrients.

The seminal vesicles are secretory glands found in the base of the prostate gland and provide the transport medium for sperm. The fluid is alkaline and contains fructose, prostaglandins, ascorbic acid and globulins.

Table 2.1 Composition of semen

Volume of ejaculate	2–6ml*
Density of spermatozoa	60–150 million/ml
Morphology	60–80% normal shape
Motility	50% should be motile after incubation for 1 hour at 37°C

Notes:
Semen or seminal fluid consists of spermatozoa and secretions from the bulbo-urethral glands and seminal vesicles, and the prostate gland.
* Values outside these normal ranges indicate infertility.

The prostate gland is found in the neck of the bladder. In an adult it is 3cm in diameter and contains mucosal glands. Prostatic secretions are thin and milky, and contain enzymes which include acid phosphatase, acid hydrolase, protease, fibrinolysin and calcium and citrates. Prostrate secretions are important for stimulating sperm motility and for neutralizing vaginal acidity.

The bulbo-urethral glands secrete mucus to provide lubrication during ejaculation; they are found between the prostate and the penis.

MALE HORMONES

Three hormones are the principal regulators of the male reproductive system; these are the hypothalamic hormones, anterior pituitary hormones and testicular hormones. Anterior pituitary hormones control spermatogenesis and androgen production and these are called **follicle-stimulating hormone** or **luteinizing hormone.**

Follicle-stimulating hormone (FSH) stimulates spermatogenesis by acting on the seminiferous tubules.

Luteinizing hormone (LH), also known as **interstitial cell-stimulating hormone (ICSH),** is required for completion of spermatogenesis by stimulating production of androgens in the interstitial cells of the Leydig.

Testosterone stimulates the development of male secondary sex characteristics and spermatogenesis. Ninety-five per cent of testosterone is synthesized and stored in the interstitial cells in the testes and 5 per cent is produced in the adrenal glands. Testosterone is synthesized from cholesterol and total adult male levels are 12 to 30nmol 1^{-1}. It is circulated in the plasma targeting reproductive organs and somatic tissues which produces the male physique, stimulates epiphyseal growth, growth of facial and body hair, libido, lowering of voice, increase in sebum secretion and mild electrolyte retention. Testosterone is metabolized and excreted by the liver.

Inhibin is thought to be produced by the sertoli cells in response to FSH stimulation and exerts a negative feedback on FSH release.

PRODUCTION OF SPERM

Production of sperm is called **spermatogenesis** and it happens in the seminiferous tubules in the testes. The seminiferous tubules are surrounded by connective tissue containing Leydig cells (interstitial cells) which are responsible for synthesis and the production of male hormones. In the seminiferous tubules there are **germ cells** and **sertoli cells**. Some of the germ cells mature to become **primary spermatocytes**. The primary spermatocytes undergo meiotic division to become **secondary spermatocytes**. These then undergo further meiotic division to become **spermatids**. Spermatids transform into **spermatozoa** with the support from sertoli cells to which they are attached; it is thought that sertoli cells help with the nutrition of germ cells. Once the spermatozoa have been produced they are released from sertoli cells into the **lumen** of the seminiferous tubules. It takes between 70 and 100 days for production of mature sperm.

Once the spermatozoa are fully formed they are pushed along the seminiferous tubules into the head of the epididymis. The tail of the epididymis is the main storage area for spermatozoa. A storage area is important as the process of spermatogenesis is continuous, while ejaculations occurs at intervals, so the spematozoa needs a storage area until it is needed, which may be up to 42 days. If ejaculation does not occur the spermatozoa degenerates. Mature spermatozoa move from the epididymis into the vas deferens and joins the seminal vesicle and the **ejaculatory duct**. The vas deferens is made up of connective tissue and three layers of smooth muscle and autonomic nerve supply. This gives the vas deferens the ability to contract quickly during ejaculation. It is this peristaltic wave and spematozoa's ability to swim that allows sperm to be released through the urethra during ejaculation.

FEMALE REPRODUCTION SYSTEM

There are 400 ova released over a female's reproductive life of 30 to 40 years. Menarche is the commencement of the menstrual cycle and usually starts at around the age of 12 to 13 but can be between 9 and 17 years. The production of ova occurs in the **ovaries**, of which there are two. The ovaries have an irregular outer

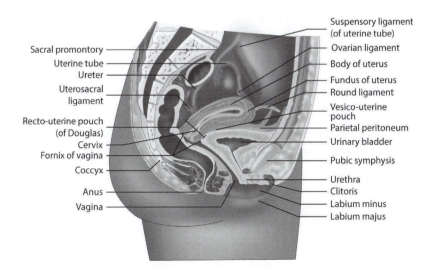

Figure 2.4 Sagital section of the female reproductive organs

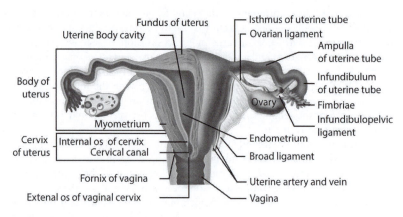

Figure 2.5 Internal female reproductive system

shape and are 4cm long, 2cm wide and 1cm thick. The outer surface is made up of columnar cells called **germinal epithelium**. The next layer is called the tunica albuginea made up of fibrous connective tissue. This layer is followed by the cortex where female germ cells are located. Female germ cells become oocytes. Finally, the inner layer is called the **vascular medulla**.

Follicles are developing oocyte and follicular tissue. The **primordial follicle** comprises cuboidal cells and these divide to form **granulosa cells**. Outside the follicle the interstitial cells change and become the **theca folliculi**, and the inner layer of this produces **oestrogens**. The follicle increases in size and becomes the **secondary follicle**. The secondary follicle matures and the granulosa cells split to form the **corona radiata** around the oocyte and the outer layer forms the **membrane granulosa**. This becomes the **Graafian follicle** which moves the surface of the ovary. A mature ovum develops within the follicle, the primordial germ cells differentiate into oogonia and, by 12 weeks of intrauterine life, they have undergone mitotic division to produce primary oocytes.

Ovulation is the release of the ovum from the Graafian follicle; it is thought that the follicular fluid pressure increases, so causing the release of the ovum. Inhibin has been found in follicular fluid and it is thought that this may determine how many follicles are released at ovulation and may have links with polycystic ovary disease. Anovulation occurs in 10 per cent of ovarian cycles, but if women have regular menstrual cycles this indicates ovulation. Some women experience lower abdominal pain on ovulation which is known as mittelschmerz, and some may experience a small amount of bleeding which is due to falling hormone levels.

The collapsed follicle becomes the **corpus luteum** which secretes oestrogen and progesterone for maintaining a pregnancy if this occurs until 12 weeks, after which time the placenta takes over this role. If there is no pregnancy the corpus luteum will degenerate after 12 to 14 days, becoming the **corpus albicans**. If fertilization occurs it happens in the ampulla of the **fallopian tube** or **uterine tube**. Only one spermatozoa can enter one ovum. There are two uterine tubes that lie within the folds of the **broad ligament**; each tube is 10 to 15cm in length and is divided into four parts.

The interstitial portion joins the wall of the uterus, while the **isthmus** is next and slightly wider, followed by the ampulla, which is the widest part of the uterine tube and where fertilization occurs, and finally by the **infundibulum**, which is trumpet shaped and has fimbria that are attached to the ovary. The uterine tube has three layers; it is covered by the **peritoneum**, and has a thin **muscular layer** followed by a **serous layer** of ciliated columnar epithelium which wafts the ovum from the infundibulum to the uterus. This serous layer has many folds called plicae and goblet-shaped cells which produce secretions to provide nutrition to the ovum.

The fertilized ovum enters the **uterus** five to six days after ovulation and four days after fertilization, and embeds in the endometrium where it will continue to grow and develop as the foetus. The uterus is pear shaped and consists of two parts: the corpus or **body** and the **cervix**. The body comprises the upper two-thirds and is 5cm long, and is usually anteverted and anteflexed, which means it tilts forward. The **fundus** is the uppermost rounded aspect of the uterus, and lies above where the uterine tubes are inserted; this area is called the **cornua**. The isthmus is 7mm long and is situated at the junction of the uterus and the cervix. The wall of the uterus is made up of three layers: the inner layer is the **endometrium,** the middle muscular layer is called the **myometrium** and the outer cover of the peritoneum is called the **perimetrium**. The uterus has three important functions: first, to receive the ovum; second, to provide an environment for the growth and development of the foetus, and finally to expel the foetus and placenta when the pregnancy is complete.

The cervix is at the lowest end of the uterus and is 2.5cm in length while the lower end projects into the vagina. In the cavity of the cervix there is an **internal os** which communicates to the uterus and the **external os** which communicates to the vagina.

The **vagina** is a fibromuscular tube which is directed backwards and upwards; it extends from the cervix to the vulva and has the ability to expand to allow a fully grown foetus through. The anterior wall of the vagina is shorter and 7.5cm in length, while the posterior wall is longer and 10cm in length. The vagina is kept

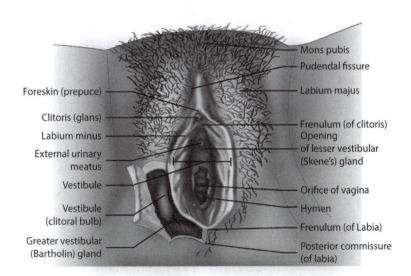

Figure 2.6 External female genitalia

lubricated by secretions from the cervical glands and transudation of serous fluid from blood-vessels on the surface. The vaginal fluid has a pH of 4.5 which contains lactic acid, and this is produced by lactobacilli working on the glycogen in the squamous cells of the vaginal lining. This lactic aid helps destroy any bacteria which enter the vagina.

The vagina opens to the vaginal orifice or introitus and the **external genitalia.** The vaginal orifice lies between the labia minora and the urethra and is partially occluded by the **hymen.** The hymen is a thin membrane, and in a virgin – someone who has not had sexual intercourse – it is intact and has a small opening. Following first sexual intercourse this is ruptured, and after vaginal delivery it is torn further, leaving a small amount of tissue, and is known as carunculae myrtiformes. **Bartholin's glands** lie on either side of the vagina and open into the vaginal canal, and their secretions, along with **Skene's glands,** lubricate the vulva, and are increased in response to the erection of the **clitoris,** helping to facilitate vaginal intercourse. Skene's glands are located behind the **urethral meatus.** The urethral meatus is the opening below the clitoris from where the urethral canal begins. The **vestibule** is the area which contains the vagina and urethra, and is only seen when the **labia minora** is separated. The clitoris is 2.5cm long and contains erectile tissue, and is found at the junction of the labia minora. It contains two erectile bodies:

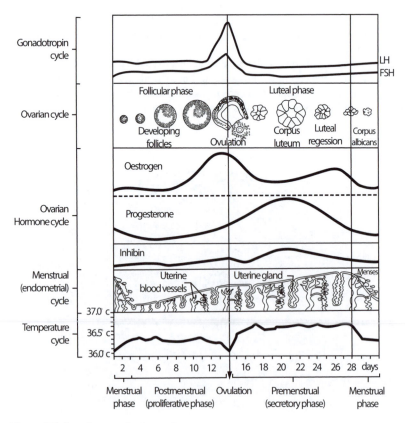

Figure 2.7 Female reproductive cycle

the **corpora cavernosa** and the **glans clitoris** which when stimulated become erect and fill with blood, just like the penis. Labia minora are two folds of skin which encircle the clitoris, forming a **hood** or **prepuce**, and then divide to enclose the vestibule, and finish as a thin fold of skin known as the **fourchette**. The **labia majora** are two thick folds of fatty tissue which extend from the **mons veneris** to the perineal body. The inner surface is smooth and the outer surface is covered by hair. The mons veneris is a pad of fat over the pubic bone and is covered by skin and hair.

It is important for health professionals to know what normal external genitalia look like and that, when a woman is examined vaginally, this area is observed to ensure that any abnormalities are detected.

The menstrual cycle is usually 28 days but may vary between 21 and 35 days. It is divided into the follicular and luteal phases. The follicular phase is when the follicle matures and ruptures, and the luteal phase is the formation of the corpus luteum, its development and degeneration.

FEMALE HORMONES

There are four main hormones which are the principal regulators of the female reproductive system.

1 *Follicle-stimulating hormone* (FSH) stimulates follicle development and oestrogen production.
2 *Luteinizing hormone* (LH) stimulates the release of the ovum.
3 *Oestrogen* prepares the body and uterus for ovulation and pregnancy. It is responsible for the growth of body, sex organs and secondary sex character-istics, prepares the endometrium for pregnancy, and makes cervical mucus thinner and more alkaline.
4 *Progesterone* prepares the body for pregnancy by maintaining the endometrium when pregnancy occurs. It stimulates the development of lobules and alveoli in the mammary glands. Premenstrual water retention is attributed to pro-gesterone and it causes a slight rise in basal body temperature during luteal phase following ovulation.

Following menstruation there are low levels of oestrogen. The hypothalamus detects this and increases **Gonadotrophin releasing hormone**, which causes **FSH** to be increased. FSH stimulates follicle development, which increases oestrogen production. The higher levels of oestrogen are detected by the hypothalamus, which reduces FSH levels. Oestrogen then prepares the uterus and body for ovulation. Because of the high levels of oestrogen there is a positive feedback to the hypo-thalamus, whereupon LH (luteinizing hormone) is produced, and **ovulation** occurs. The corpus luteum forms from the collapsed follicle after ovulation and secretes progesterone and oestrogen; these stop gonadotrophins and prepare the body for pregnancy. If the ovum is not fertilized, the corpus luteum degenerates, hormone levels drop and menstruation occurs.

The menstrual cycle

The menstrual cycle describes the changes to the endometrium. The menstrual cycle is usually 28 days in length but may vary between 21 and 35 days. The menstrual cycle is divided into three stages:

1 **Proliferative phase** lasts 10 to 11 days and coincides with ovarian follicle growth and secretion of oestrogen. The endometrium gradually builds up.
2 **Secretory phase** lasts 14 days and is under the influence of progesterone and oestrogen. The endometrium is now 5mm thick. If after 12 to 14 days no fertilization has taken place the corpus luteum will degenerate and oestrogen and progesterone decline, resulting in menstruation.
3 **Menstrual phase** lasts three to seven days and is where menses occur, at the end of which the endometrium will be 0.5mm thick.

SEXUAL INTERCOURSE

Both men and women experience the sexual response cycle during sexual intercourse. This follows four phases: **Desire, Excitement, Plateau, Orgasm** and **Resolution**. Desire is influenced through stimuli that may be from many different areas, such as environment or culture, and causes the initiation of or receptiveness to sexual activity. Excitement develops through stimulation. Plateau is a consolidation period in which intense stimulation will be intensified. Orgasm is where there are involuntary contractions, causing the peaking of sexual pleasure and the release in sexual tension. Resolution is where the body returns to its pre-excitement state which may be seen in loss of erection or the decrease in the clitoris's size, and vasocongestion is relieved. If orgasm does not occur then discomfort in the genital area may be experienced as vasocongestion has not been relieved.

The sexual response cycle can be influenced by cultural, religious and personal experiences. Communication between sexual partners is a vital aspect of satisfying sexual intercourse; however, this is not always an area that people feel confident to discuss with their sexual partners and so can lead to loss of libido, failure to achieve orgasm or premature ejaculation. Psychosexual counselling of the individual or couple can address psychological causes and is available through referral in most sexual health services.

THE MALE

When a man is aroused the penis becomes erect through the dilatation of arterioles in corpus spongiosum and corpora cavernosa, the erectile tissue inside the penis. The arterioles dilate and become engorged with blood, and the penis becomes enlarged in length and width. An erection can occur through direct stimulation, or from thought, visual or emotional material; it is controlled by spinal reflex. The erection reflex can begin with the stimulation of highly sensitive mechanoreceptors at the tip of the penis. The afferent synapse in the lower spinal cord and the efferent flow via the nervi erigentes produce relaxation in the arterioles in the corpus spongiosum and corpora cavernosa. At the same time parasympathetic nerves stimulate the urethral glands to produce a secretion to aid lubrication, and entry of the erect penis into the vagina. Following ejaculation a man will experience a refractory period in which he is unable to ejaculate further, although he may be capable of partial erection.

THE FEMALE

When a woman is sexually excited the clitoris and the labia minora will become erect, the breasts will enlarge and the nipples become erect. The vagina will become lubricated and this will aid vaginal penetration by the penis. Women achieve orgasm through the stimulation of the clitoris and the cervix, and they are able to achieve several orgasms within a short period of time. Orgasm causes the cervix and uterus to contract rhythmically, aiding the aspiration of sperm into the uterus, but orgasm is not necessary for fertilization. Women do not have a refractory period so may be able to experience repeated orgasms before reaching resolution.

THE EFFECT OF AGE ON MEN AND WOMEN

Menopause usually occurs in women between the ages of 45 and 55, while the mean age in the UK is 48 years. The menopause is the permanent cessation of menses with loss of ovarian function. It is defined as 12 months of no menstruation, which can only be diagnosed retrospectively. During the menopause there is a deficiency of oestrogen and progesterone. The hypothalamus responds by increasing gonadotrophins, follicle-stimulating hormone and luteinizing hormone which may be 10 times the level found in a normal menstruating woman. The reduction of oestrogen and progesterone and increase of follicle-stimulating and luteinizing hormones result in menopausal symptoms. Menopausal symptoms can vary among women, but women can complain of vaginal dryness, hot flushes and headaches. Women under the age of 50 should use contraception for two years after their last menstrual period, and women over the age of 50 should be advised to use contraception for one year after their last period (FSRH, 2010c).

From the age of 55 or older, men tend to have less firm erections, produce smaller amounts of semen and experience less intense ejaculations, with less need to ejaculate and a longer resolution period. Erectile dysfunction in men under the age of 40 is likely to be caused by psychological issues. However, in men over 40 who experience erectile dysfunction, this can be a warning sign of hidden medical problems such as diabetes, hypertension or raised cholesterol.

In two out of three men with hypertension, erectile dysfunction is experienced. Just as the coronary arteries to the heart can be occluded with atheroma, so can the arteries to the penis, causing problems with erections. Men should be encouraged to keep their weight and cholesterol within normal limits, not to smoke and keep fit not just for their heart but also for a healthy sex life.

FURTHER READING

If you interested in this area and would like further information, you may find the following websites useful.

Sexual Advice Association: www.sda.uk.net.
British Society for Sexual Medicine: www.bssm.org.uk.

3

NATURAL FAMILY PLANNING METHODS: FERTILITY AWARENESS

- Introduction
- History
- Explanation of the method
- Efficacy
- Disadvantages of natural family planning methods
- Advantages of natural family planning methods
- The temperature method
- The cervical mucus method
- The calendar method
- Combination of methods
- The personal contraceptive system
- Lactational amenorrhoea method
- The future
- Sexuality and anxieties

INTRODUCTION

Natural family planning methods have been used widely in the past by various religious groups such as the Roman Catholic faith. They involve the observation of certain body changes which denote ovulation. From this information a couple may choose to either abstain from sexual intercourse and use it as their family planning method, or use this fertile period to have sexual intercourse promoting pregnancy, known as fertility awareness.

HISTORY

Natural family planning methods have been referred to previously as periodic abstinence, the safe period and the rhythm method. It is only more recently that it has been promoted to women as a fertility awareness method, and as more women are delaying pregnancy this has become a popular choice. Infertility clinics may ask women at initial consultations to use fertility awareness kits; previously they used the temperature method to indicate ovulation.

In 1930 Ogino in Japan and in 1933 Knaus in Austria found that conception took place in between menstrual cycles, and the time from ovulation to the next menstrual period was always the same regardless of the cycle. Using this information they developed the calendar method. Around this period changes in the cervical mucus were noted by Seguy and Vimeux. Ferin in 1947 first noticed that a woman's body temperature changed at ovulation. However, it was not until 1964 that Drs John and Evelyn Billings used these discoveries to formulate the Billings method, now known as the cervical method.

Recently, research has increased in this area producing personal contraceptive systems and urinary dipsticks. The temperature method has benefited from electronic and digital thermometers by increasing accuracy and decreasing the time clients need to take their temperature.

EXPLANATION OF THE METHOD

There are four main natural family planning and fertility awareness methods:

1 The temperature method.
2 The cervical mucus method (previously known as the Billings method).
3 The calendar method.
4 Combination of methods, also known as the sympto-thermal method or double-check method.

These methods help a woman recognize when ovulation takes place. This usually occurs between days 12 and 16 before the next menstrual period. The ovum remains capable of being fertilized for 12 to 24 hours, while sperm are capable of fertilizing the ovum for three to five days and on occasions have survived up to seven days *in utero* (see Fig. 3.1).

During each menstrual cycle the pituitary gland releases follicle-stimulating hormone (FSH). This triggers the development of follicles which contain the immature ova and is known as the **follicular phase**. As the follicles develop they secrete the hormone oestrogen. This causes the reduction of FSH so that further ovum development is inhibited, the endometrium becomes thickened ready for implantation, and the cervical glands produce mucus favourable to sperm penetration. As the ovum ripens the level of oestrogen rises, causing the pituitary gland to produce luteinizing hormone (LH). This causes the follicle to rupture, releasing the ovum into the fallopian tube; this is known as **ovulation**. Rising oestrogen levels cause the cervix to soften and rise upwards and the **os** to open. The empty follicle becomes the corpus luteum, which secretes the hormone progesterone. This part of the menstrual cycle is known as the **luteal phase**. Progesterone causes the basal body temperature to rise during the luteal phase after ovulation. The pituitary gland is now inhibited from producing LH and FSH so that further ovulation is prevented. Following ovulation cervical mucus becomes thickened and sticky, making sperm penetration difficult. The cervix becomes firm and the os closes. If the ovum is fertilized the corpus luteum will continue to produce progesterone throughout early pregnancy. However, if the ovum is not fertilized the corpus luteum will disintegrate, the level of progesterone will drop and menstruation will occur. The shift in basal body temperature, position of the cervix and change in cervical mucus are all used as indicators for natural family planning and fertility awareness to assess when a woman is fertile.

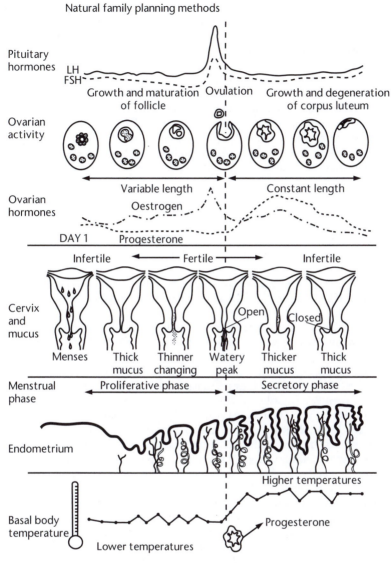

Natural family planning methods

Figure 3.1 Changes during the menstrual cycle. (Reproduced with kind permission from 'Fertility' – Fertility Awareness and Natural Family Planning, 3rd edn, E. Clubb and J. Knight, 1996, David & Charles.)

EFFICACY

The efficacy of natural family planning methods is 80 to 98 per cent with careful use. The sympto-thermal is the most effective method as it uses a combination of methods. In theory the efficacy of the sympto-thermal method can be as high as 98 per cent; however, with this and any natural family planning method the range of effectiveness of the method is dependent on the user, and is known as the user failure rate. The efficacy is dependent on the level of motivation and commitment the couple invest in the method. Many men and women use this method to space their pregnancies, and as a result may be prepared to take more risks – a pregnancy slightly earlier than planned may be a happy accident! However, couples who are using the method to avoid pregnancy are more likely to be highly motivated and conscientious; they are less likely to take risks, so the user failure rate will be lower and the efficacy higher. Finally, the level and expertise of the teaching of this method will influence its efficacy, which is why it is vital that this method is taught by a teacher trained in natural family planning. If you are interested in training in natural methods or need to refer a client to a trainer you should access the Fertility UK website on www.fertilityuk.org. This is an excellent source of information.

UKMEC

UKMEC use different categories to give advice on fertility awareness based on methods that should be used. These are as follows:

- *Accept*: There is no medical reason to deny the use of fertility awareness-based methods if the women is not breast-feeding and more than four weeks post-partum.
- *Caution*: The method is normally provided in a routine setting with extra preparation and precautions. For fertility awareness methods this means counselling may be needed to ensure correct use of the method (FSRH, 2009a). Caution should be taken by women who are in the first two-year post-menarche and peri-menopause, or in breast-feeding women who are over six weeks post-partum or after menses begin.
- *Delay*: Use of the method should be delayed until the condition is evaluated or changes (FSRH, 2009a). Fertility awareness methods should be delayed with women breast-feeding within six weeks post-partum and within four weeks post-partum in non-breast-feeding women, and post-abortion. This is because there will not be sufficient ovarian function for detectable fertility signs. Fertility awareness methods should be delayed if there is any vaginal discharge or irregular bleeding. Certain medications such as Lithium, antidepressants, anti-anxiety and some antibiotics and anti-inflammatory drugs may alter the menstrual cycle or affect fertility signs such as cervical mucus, making it not possible to use fertility awareness or personal contraceptives as methods.

DISADVANTAGES OF NATURAL FAMILY PLANNING METHODS

- Requires motivation.
- Needs to be taught by a specialist in natural family planning.
- Requires the observation and recording of changes in the body.
- May take time to learn so may require a period of abstinence.

- Once learnt it is under the control of the couple.
- Inexpensive (except in the personal contraceptive method).
- May be used to promote pregnancy.
- Increases couple's knowledge of changes in the body and fertility.
- No physical side effects.
- Acceptable to some religious beliefs and cultures.

THE TEMPERATURE METHOD

The temperature method involves the woman taking her temperature every day to record her basal body temperature. Following ovulation the basal body temperature (BBT) will drop slightly and then rise by 0.2 to 0.4°C where it will stay until the next period. This occurs because following ovulation the hormone progesterone is secreted by the corpus luteum which causes a woman's basal body temperature to rise (see Fig. 3.2).

The client should be advised to take her temperature at the same time each day before getting out of bed. If she works night shifts she should do this after waking in the evening. She should take her temperature first before drinking or eating, as these will affect the basal body temperature. The thermometer should be an ovulation thermometer which is calibrated in tenths of a degree between the range of 35 and 39°C. A digital or electronic thermometer may be used which takes about 45 seconds to give a reading. The temperature can be taken orally which takes five minutes, or vaginally or rectally which takes three minutes. The temperature should always be taken by the same route to avoid inaccuracy. The temperature is recorded on a chart commencing on the first day of her menstrual period (see Fig. 3.2). Once the temperature has risen and has been maintained for three days the couple may have unprotected sexual intercourse until the first day of the next menstrual period.

Disadvantages

- Requires motivation.
- Needs to be taught by a specialist in natural family planning.
- The basal body temperature is affected by illness, disturbed sleep, stress, alcohol and drugs (e.g. aspirin).
- If the temperature is not taken at roughly the same time each day this will lead to inaccuracies in the BBT.
- Does not detect the beginning of the fertile period, making it harder to achieve pregnancy.
- Requires long periods of abstinence, as it only detects post-ovulation.

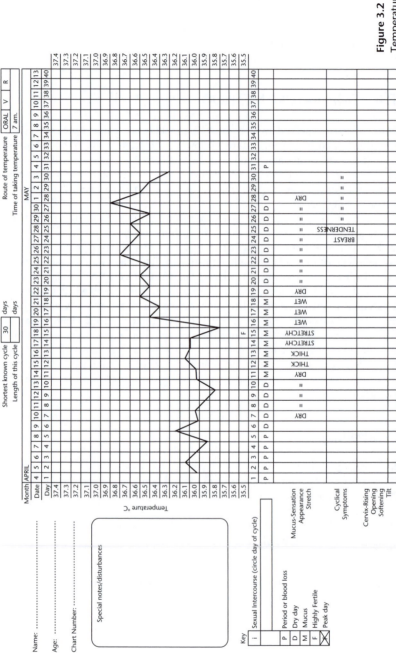

Figure 3.2
Temperature chart

Advantages

- Increases the couple's knowledge and awareness of the fertile period.
- Helpful to women who experience erratic cycles by detecting ovulation.
- Can help to pinpoint other body changes such as cervical mucus.
- Under the woman's control.
- May be used to prevent or promote pregnancy.

THE CERVICAL MUCUS METHOD

The cervical mucus method involves a woman observing her cervical mucus every day. The mucus varies throughout the cycle. Following menstruation there is little cervical mucus and this is often described as 'dry'. The level of the hormones oestrogen and progesterone are low and the mucus is known as infertile mucus. There may be an absence of cervical mucus or it may appear sticky and, if stretched between two fingers, will break. As the ovum begins to ripen, increasing amounts of oestrogen are produced, causing an increase in cervical mucus. This marks the beginning of the fertile phase. Oestrogen levels continue to rise prior to ovulation and the cervical mucus increases in amount, becoming clear and stretchy; if held between two fingers it can stretch easily without breaking. It has been described

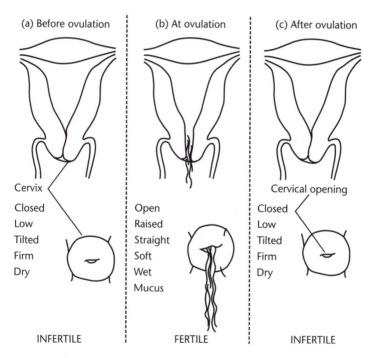

Figure 3.3 Changes in the cervix during the menstrual cycle. (Reproduced with kind permission from 'Fertility' – Fertility Awareness and Natural Family Planning, 3rd edn, E. Clubb and J. Knight, 1996, David & Charles)

as resembling raw egg white and is called fertile mucus. The last day of this type of mucus is known as peak mucus day; which can only be identified retrospectively. Four days following peak mucus day the mucus becomes thick, sticky and opaque, and is known as infertile mucus. This change in the mucus occurs because the ovum has been released and the level of oestrogen has dropped (see Fig. 3.3).

The woman is taught to observe and record her cervical mucus several times a day either by collecting some on toilet paper or by inserting her fingers into her vagina to check its consistency and appearance. She will also be encouraged to become aware of changes in sensation of her cervical mucus. Trials (Indian Council of Medical Research Task Force on Natural Family Planning, 1996) looking at the cervical mucus method have shown a method failure rate of 1.5 per 100 users and a user failure rate of the method of 15.9 per 100 users at 21 months. This would seem to illustrate how vital training and motivation of the client and her partner are in ensuring efficacy.

Disadvantages

- Requires commitment.
- Needs to be taught by a specialist in natural family planning.
- Can take two to three cycles to learn method.
- Vaginal infections can make it difficult to identify fertile mucus.
- Some drugs used for treatment of colds, etc. can inhibit cervical mucus production.
- Involves touching the body which some women may dislike.
- Requires abstinence.

Advantages

- Under the control of the woman.
- Gives the couple permission to touch their bodies.
- Increases awareness of body changes.
- Predicts fertile mucus, thus enabling pregnancy.
- May be used to prevent pregnancy.

THE CALENDAR METHOD

The calendar method involves a woman detecting when her fertile period is, which is usually 12 to 16 days before the first day of her next menstrual period. This is based on looking retrospectively at the woman's menstrual cycle for a period of 6 to 12 months of recorded cycles. This method is no longer recognized as reliable on its own, but may be taught alongside another method as in the combination of methods.

Disadvantages

- Unreliable, as it does not take into account irregular cycles.
- Stress, illness and travelling can affect the menstrual cycle.

■ Requires motivation.
■ Requires menstrual cycle to be recorded for 6 to 12 months prior to use.

Advantages

■ Under the control of the woman.
■ Increases knowledge about fertility.
■ May be used in conjunction with another method.

COMBINATION OF METHODS

This is often referred to as the sympto-thermal method or double-check method and combines the temperature, calendar and cervical mucus methods, which is why it is more effective as a contraceptive. Women are also encouraged to observe changes in their cervix such as consistency, position, and whether their cervical os is open or closed. During the beginning of the cycle when the levels of oestrogen and progesterone are reduced, the cervix is positioned low in the vagina and can be easily felt. The cervical os is closed, and the cervix feels firm to the touch. As oestrogen levels increase the cervix changes and at peak mucus day feels soft. The os is now open and the cervix has risen higher into the vagina, making it harder to locate. Following ovulation the cervix returns to its former state, positioned lower, and feels firmer with the os closed. Checking the position and consistency of the cervix, along with the cervical mucus method, can easily be performed by either partner. Women are encouraged to observe and record mood changes and breast tenderness which usually occur in the latter part of the cycle. She may be aware of ovulation pain (known as **mittelschmerz**) and/or mid-cycle bleeding. All these indicators help to confirm changes in the cycle.

Disadvantages

■ Requires motivation.
■ Needs to be taught by a specialist in natural family planning.
■ Requires daily commitment.

Advantages

■ Detects beginning and end of fertile phase.
■ May be used to promote pregnancy.
■ Higher contraceptive efficacy than any other single natural family planning method.

SELF-ASSESSMENT QUESTIONS

Answers and discussion at the end of the chapter.

1   What sorts of problems with the natural family planning method do you think your client may encounter?
2   How would you help your clients solve these problems?
3   For whom do you think this method might be unsuitable and why?

THE PERSONAL CONTRACEPTIVE SYSTEM

Persona is the first personal contraceptive system, under the control of the woman, which identifies when a woman is fertile. With careful and consistent use Persona is between 93 and 97 per cent effective in preventing pregnancy. Prospective research on efficacy and acceptability has found Persona to be 93.8 per cent effective in preventing pregnancy when abstinence is used during the identified fertile period (Bonnar *et al.*, 1999) (Fig. 3.4).

Persona monitors (through a database) luteinizing hormone and oestrone-3-glucuronide (a metabolite of oestradiol). By testing her urine through urinary test sticks, information is given to the woman's database which is interpreted, telling

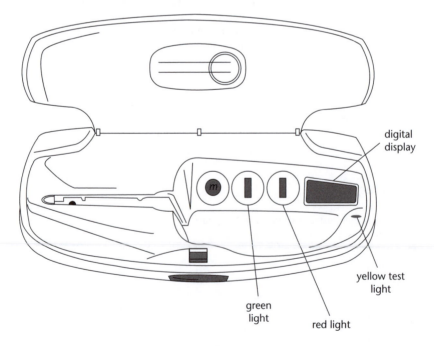

digital display

yellow test light

green light

red light

Figure 3.4 Showing operation. (Reproduced with kind permission of Unipath Ltd)

her whether she is fertile or not. Persona tells a woman when the fertile period commences and ends through a system of lights: a green light indicates she is safe to have sexual intercourse; a red light indicates she should abstain or use a barrier method of contraception (this is usually 6 to 10 days each cycle). A yellow light indicates that she should perform a urine test to give the database more information. A urine test should be performed on an early morning urine sample and then inserted into the machine. Usually this needs to be performed 8 days a month, but in the first month it will need to be done 16 days of the month to provide the database with information about the woman.

Persona may be bought over the counter for the starter pack or online from www.persona.info/uk at a cost of £64.95 plus p&p and a further £9.95 each month for test sticks. A care line has been instituted by Unipath for women with fully trained staff on persona so that advice may be given about any problems she has with this method. The telephone line is open 7 a.m. to 6 p.m. weekdays and 9 a.m. to 12 midday at weekends.

Disadvantages

■ Expensive.
■ May only be used by women whose menstrual cycle falls within the range of 23 to 35 days.
■ Does not protect against sexually transmitted diseases or **human immunodeficiency virus** (HIV).

Advantages

■ No systemic effects.
■ Under the control of the woman.
■ May be used to plan pregnancy.
■ Easily reversed.

Absolute contra-indications

■ Not suitable for women whose menstrual cycle does not fall in the range of 23 to 35 days.
■ Not suitable for women who are breast-feeding.
■ Not suitable for women using hormone treatments.
■ Not suitable for women with kidney or liver disease.
■ Not suitable for women with menopausal symptoms.
■ Not suitable for women with polycystic ovarian syndrome.

LACTATIONAL AMENORRHOEA METHOD (LAM)

The Lactational Amenorrhoea Method is the use of breast-feeding to inhibit ovulation and act as a contraceptive. If a woman has a baby of under 6 months old and is amenorrhoeic and fully breast-feeding there is only about a 2 per cent chance of pregnancy occurring. However, if a woman is not fully breast-feeding or not amenorrhoeic the risk of pregnancy will be greater. Many women will choose to rely on another method of contraception such as barrier methods or the progestogen-only pill as well as LAM.

One of the difficulties with this method is that women in the Western world are encouraged and motivated to stop night-time feeding and this may not give sufficient stimulation to inhibit ovulation.

CASE STUDY 3.1

A 51-year-old woman consulted having used natural family planning all her fertile life. She had used no other contraceptive method and had had three planned pregnancies. She was finding it difficult to identify when ovulation was occurring and was finding long periods of abstinence unsatisfactory.

Following discussion with the woman, she agreed that she and her partner would use condoms and she would continue with natural family planning. She decided that a diaphragm would stop her being able to use the natural family planning method, as the use of a spermicide would affect the detection of changes in the cervical mucus.

SELF-ASSESSMENT QUESTIONS

Answers and discussion at the end of the chapter.

4 Which day of a woman's menstrual cycle is counted as the first day?
5 If a woman has a regular cycle of 5/35 days, when is she most likely to be fertile?
6 If a woman has a regular cycle of 3/21 days, when is she most likely to be fertile?

THE FUTURE

New innovations in natural family planning have focused on making the methods accessible to women. The Standard Days method uses the knowledge of fertility awareness methods to identify the fertile window of days 8 to 19 of the cycle and avoid unprotected sexual intercourse (Sinai *et al.*, 2012). These methods are particularly useful in countries where contraception is limited, as seen in research undertaken in Ethiopia (Bekele and Fantahun, 2012). Cyclebeads were used in Ethiopia to illustrate the Standard Days method; these are a string of beads which represent each day of the cycle: they are coloured white or brown; white beads indicate days when you can get pregnant and brown beads are days when you are not likely to get pregnant. The Standard Days method is advocated for women with cycles of 26 to 32 days. This method offers important solutions to women throughout the world; it is inexpensive and easy to use, and within the control of the woman.

Women who choose natural family planning methods as a contraceptive or as a means of becoming pregnant can find this method empowering; it gives them control of their lives and gives information about their body that is often concealed from them. As a method it gives men and women permission to investigate and touch a woman's body. Sometimes when a woman tries this method she finds that her cycle is not as regular as she first thought, leading to longer periods of abstinence than initially anticipated (Flynn, 1996). However, it may be argued that periodic abstinence can enhance a relationship, giving a woman and her partner time to enjoy a non-penetrative sexual relationship, creating greater understanding of each other (Ryder and Campbell, 1995).

For women who choose this method it can be empowering; freedom of choice allows this. However, for some women, whether for moral or religious reasons this is the only acceptable method; this can feel very limiting and unsatisfactory. If a woman has experienced unwanted or several pregnancies there may be anxiety about becoming pregnant again in the future, and it may be a good time to discuss this method and whether another method may be more suitable.

If either member of the couple has anxieties with this method – perhaps a partner does not want another pregnancy, or if it is used as a means of promoting pregnancy then a partner may feel a pressure to 'perform' – this may manifest itself with sexual dysfunction. Some male clients who feel a pressure to 'perform' may complain of loss of libido or erectile problems. Women who are anxious about becoming pregnant may complain of loss of libido and lack of sexual enjoyment. These problems may be very difficult for the client to discuss, but it is important that during the consultation you listen to the feelings in yourself that are evoked by the consultation (e.g. anger, sadness), as these will help you try to understand how your client feels about the situation and whether they may wish to be referred for psychosexual counselling.

ANSWERS TO SELF-ASSESSMENT QUESTIONS

1   *What sorts of problems with the natural family planning method do you think your client may encounter?*

Your client may encounter problems locating her cervix or may find it difficult to distinguish between the changes in the cervical mucus. She may find it difficult to remember to take her temperature every day at the same time, especially if she has young children or works shifts.

If she is unwell or has had a disturbed sleep pattern this will affect her basal body temperature. Events like late-night parties, children waking in the night and alcohol consumption will all affect the BBT. If your client's cycle has been affected by a change in hormone levels and she has secondary amenorrhoea, for example, following pregnancy or at the menopause, she may find it difficult to interpret her fertile phase, and another method may be more appropriate.

2   *How would you solve these problems?*

If your client has difficulty locating her cervix then she will need to be taught. She may find it easier to feel her cervix if she uses a squatting position or in a standing position with one foot on a chair, and if she tries feeling during her infertile phase when the cervix is lower and easier to feel.

If there are problems distinguishing between the changes in the cervical mucus it is important to eliminate vaginal infection which would camouflage normal discharge. Your client may lack confidence in and knowledge of her mucus changes; it may be a good idea to book more frequent consultations so that you can check the cervical mucus together throughout her cycle.

Difficulty remembering temperature taking may be solved with an alarm. A digital thermometer may be useful as it only takes 45 seconds to record the temperature, and if a mother is rushing out of bed for a crying child this may be a suitable compromise. The problem may signify the woman's dissatisfaction with the method, and another method may be more suitable.

3   *For whom do you think this method might be unsuitable and why?*

Women who have a delay in ovulation caused by secondary amenorrhoea following childbirth or the menopause would need to have long periods of abstinence, which makes this method unsuitable for these women.

Other women who would be considered unsuitable for this method are women who do not want to get pregnant and require a contraceptive with a high efficacy. The method would be unsuitable for women where pregnancy would be detrimental to their health or that of the foetus (e.g. following administration of a live vaccine when teratogenesis is a risk).

4   *Which day of a woman's menstrual cycle is counted as the first day?*

The first day of a woman's menstrual cycle is counted as the first day of her period. Many women think that the first day of their cycle is at the end of their period.

5   *If a woman has a regular menstrual cycle of 5/35 days, when is she most likely to be fertile?*

A woman ovulates between 12 and 16 days before her next period; therefore a woman with a regular 35-day cycle would be fertile between days 19 and 23 of her cycle.

6   *If a woman has a regular menstrual cycle of 3/21 days, when is she most likely to be fertile?*

A woman with a regular 21-day cycle would be fertile between days 5 and 8 of her cycle.

SEXUALLY TRANSMITTED INFECTIONS

4

- Introduction
- History
- Taking a sexual history
- Screening for STIs in asymptomatic men and women
- Screening for STIs in symptomatic men and women
- Symptomatic women
- Symptomatic men
- Types of sexually transmitted infections
- Non-sexually transmitted infections
- Sexuality and anxieties

INTRODUCTION

Sexual intercourse is a fundamental part of being human, but with it arises risks. Much of this book focuses on avoiding unwanted pregnancies; however, a huge risk of sexual intercourse is sexually transmitted infections (STIs). There are many views about sexually transmitted infections; many men and women believe that they are not at risk, some will see it as 'par for the course' and others will be horrified. But whatever views they hold, STIs have a huge psychological and emotional impact alone, without adding in the repercussions for fertility.

HISTORY

Syphilis is documented as early as the fifteenth century and was known as the great pox because of its long incubation period; it was not associated with sexual intercourse for some time. In the eighteenth century, it was known that syphilis and gonorrhoea were venereal diseases. In 1916, during the First World War when there was an increase in the incidence of syphilis and gonorrhoea, a Royal Commission on Venereal Diseases set up a network of national clinics to help treat the problem. The second surge of STIs occurred following the Second World War and in 1948 the National Health Service took over these clinics.

Today, these clinics are known as sexual health clinics and are increasingly integrated with contraception to provide both services. Information in sexual health clinics is anonymized to maintain confidentiality, and is not disclosed without a client's consent to their general practitioner; every effort is made to ensure that patients' confidentiality is maintained to encourage men and women to attend.

TAKING A SEXUAL HISTORY

When commencing your consultation, you will want to discuss confidentiality and, throughout your session, you will want to ascertain also whether this is consenting sexual intercourse, whether the person is under 18 years of age and needs to be assessed for child protection risks or whether they are a vulnerable adult. Your client may have been sexually assaulted and you should be watching for anything that gives you concern that this has occurred so that you can tailor your care around this knowledge.

When taking a sexual history it is important to find out what has brought the person to the clinic: are they anxious about a particular episode of sexual intercourse or a rash, for example? This will also help when you cover the issue of window periods for sexually transmitted infections, as the episode may/may not be covered and the client may have to repeat the screening.

You will also need to know whether your client is taking any other medications, their medical history and whether they are allergic to anything. If the client is a woman, you will need to know when her last menstrual period was, so that you can eliminate pregnancy or perform a pregnancy test if indicated. You will also need to know what form of contraception the woman uses.

You will then need to ask whether they have any symptoms; if they are asymptomatic you can perform an asymptomatic screen. If they have any of the symptoms described in Table 4.1 they will need to examined.

It is useful to find out how long your client has had the symptoms, whether they have worsened. If they have pain, does it come and go, or is it there all the time? What makes the pain worse? If your client is a woman you should consider performing a pregnancy test, as this could be an ectopic pregnancy or pelvic inflammatory disease (PID).

It is also important to ask whether your client has had any sexually transmitted infections. If so, when was this and where were they treated? If it was recently, it

Table 4.1 STI symptoms in men and women

Symptoms for men	Symptoms for women
Discharge from penis	Discharge from vagina which is different from normal
Dysuria – pain or discomfort passing urine	Dysuria – pain or discomfort passing urine
Frequency of micturition	Frequency of micturition
Testicular pain	Abdominal pain
Rashes, lumps or sores in genital area	Rashes, lumps or sores in genital area
Discharge/bleeding from anus	Abnormal vaginal bleeding, post-coital bleeding
	Discharge/ bleeding from anus
	Dyspareunia

is possible that they may still have the infection and you should consider treatment failure. This could because of:

- *Poor compliance*: patient not completing antibiotic course.
- *Re-infection*: patient not abstaining from sexual intercourse for seven days after completing treatment or having sexual intercourse with a partner who is still infected.
- *Antibiotic resistance*: most likely with gonorrhoea infections, which is why cultures are performed to ensure that an antibiotic is given to which it is sensitive.
- *Drug interaction/poor absorption*: most likely cause is vomiting within two hours of ingesting Azithromycin treatment for chlamydia, for example.

You will also need to find out about your client's sexual partners during the past three months and the type of sexual intercourse to ensure correct screening; this helps to clarify the risk of infection. This is best achieved by asking: When was the client's last sexual intercourse? Was this a male or female partner? How long have they been having sexual intercourse? What type of sexual intercourse – oral, vaginal, anal – were they having? Did they use a condom? This could be abbreviated to the following:

LSI – 2/7 cfp 3/12 vi – condom used, oi no condom

(Last sexual intercourse two days ago with casual female partner of three months, vaginal intercourse with a condom, oral intercourse, no condom used.)

You would then ask about the previous sexual partner for the previous three months:

PSP 1 – 5/7 rfp 12/12 – vi no condom used

(Previous sexual partner one, last sexual intercourse with them five days ago, regular female partner of one year, vaginal intercourse, no condom used.)

The next question would be as follows:

PSP 2 – 1/12 cmp 1/7, oi r no condom. Ai i+r condom used

(Previous sexual partners two, last sexual intercourse with them one month ago with a casual male partner one episode. Received oral sex, no condom used. Insertive and receptive anal intercourse with a condom.)

This would tell you that this male client would need rectal, oral and urethral screening, and you should discuss the risks of Hepatitis A and B as well as screening and immunization for these conditions, as he has sex with men.

It is important that you ask all clients without making assumptions about their sexuality, as that could lead to you missing someone who may be at risk. Finally, if a client requires a genital examination you should have undergone training to do this; if you are not trained to carry out these procedures you will need to refer the client to a sexual health clinic.

SCREENING FOR STIS IN ASYMPTOMATIC MEN AND WOMEN

Prior to performing any test, you should discuss what the test is for and any window period, the implications of a positive result and how the client will receive the results. Clients may choose not to screen for all STIs and may wish to have more time before considering an HIV test, for example. It is important that clients have enough information so that they are able to give their consent.

If a man or woman is asymptomatic they can be screened for chlamydia and gonorrhoea. A woman can do a vaginal self-swab; this is more sensitive in women than a urine test. A man can do a urine test and should not have passed urine for two hours. The most sensitive test for gonorrhoea and chlamydia available is a NAAT test (nucleic acid amplification test) and this will pick up infection from 14 days previously.

Blood tests for HIV and syphilis (serum treponemal serology – STS) should be discussed with all patients. Fourth-generation HIV tests are the most sensitive form of testing for HIV antibodies and P24 antigens, and are 99 to 100 per cent sensitive; they will also give the result of HIV infection from the previous four weeks. Third-generation HIV tests are still available but are not the first choice because they are less accurate. These tests have a window period of three months, meaning they will give a result from three months prior to the test; this is because they only screen for HIV antibodies which are only detectable after three months and are 98.9 per cent sensitive. You should be aware of the type of screening available in your area. HIV screening should be encouraged in all men and women, but those who are particularly at risk are those who come from geographical areas where HIV is widespread, such as sub-Saharan Africa, and specific groups, such as men who have sex with men (MSM), intravenous drug users, commercial sex workers, victims of sexual assault, needle stick injuries and people who have an existing acute episode of an STI .

In early syphilis the serology may be negative, and, if this is suspected, it should be repeated after three months. Hepatitis A IgG screening should be considered for men who have sex with men, and if this does not show any immunity to the infection they should be vaccinated. Hepatitis B core antibody screening should be considered for men who have sex with men, intravenous drug users (IVDU) and for patients who grew up in a tropical country such as China or Africa. If this is positive they will need to be referred to the Liver Unit and partners will need screening; if this is negative vaccination should be considered. Hepatitis B surface antibody is performed when previous vaccination has been done to detect the level of immunity and should be done every five years. Hepatitis C screening should be considered for intravenous drug users and men who have sex with men who are HIV positive. If serology is positive then the client will need to be referred to the Liver Unit; there is no vaccination for Hepatitis C.

SCREENING FOR STIS IN SYMPTOMATIC MEN AND WOMEN

If a person is symptomatic they will need to screened and examined. They may be expecting this, but it is important before you start that you explain what you are about to do and why you need to do it. You will need to discuss what tests you are considering doing and why, and what this will mean if they are positive, to ensure that consent is obtained. It is easy to forget the impact of a positive test on a relationship; however, it is important that clients agree to this, and understand how and when they will get the results.

You should always offer a chaperone whether the client is male or female, and ensure sufficient privacy is given during the examination.

SYMPTOMATIC WOMEN

For a symptomatic woman you should perform a pregnancy test if she has any abdominal pain or had a late or abnormal period prior to examination; if positive she will need to be seen by a doctor. A pregnancy test will give you a result from three weeks ago. If your client has any urinary symptoms you will need to perform a urinalysis and may want to send a midstream urine sample (MSU) to microbiology. If the pregnancy test is negative and she is not complaining of abdominal pain you will need to perform a speculum examination and take swabs for microbiology from the vagina and endocervix for gonorrhoea sensitivities, and a gonorrhoea and chlamydia NAAT from the endocervix. When performing a speculum examination it is good practice not to use any lubricating gel as this can obscure the sample; wetting the speculum with some warm water should be sufficient. If you are working in a sexual health clinic where microscopy is available, then a dry and wet slide will be done. The wet slide for Trichomonas and dry slide will have samples from the urethra, cervix and vagina and, once stained, this enables staff to diagnose bacterial vaginosis, candida and gonorrhoea. This helps to aid diagnosis and treatment.

If you are trained, a bimanual examination should be performed to eliminate pelvic inflammatory disease (PID). All the time you should be observing whether the vulva, vagina and cervix look normal; you are looking for anything abnormal.

Blood tests for HIV, syphilis and hepatitis should be done if required. If a woman has an ulcer in the genital area this could be genital herpes and a swab should be taken; this could also be syphilis, so serology is important to exclude this possibility.

SYMPTOMATIC MEN

A symptomatic man will need to be examined. This will include palpation of testes for lumps, and checking the groin for raised lymph nodes (normally you should be unable to feel these), since this could indicate a viral infection. You should observe the penis. Does it look normal? Is he circumcised or not? If he has a foreskin, can the client move it easily so that you can take a specimen from the urethra? If the client has problems retracting his foreskin then this should be taken seriously and he will need to be seen by a doctor, and may need to be referred to Accident and Emergency. If a man has discharge from his penis a urethral specimen should be taken for gonorrhoea sensitivities and, if microscopy is available, a dry slide. This should be followed by a urine specimen for chlamydia and gonorrhoea NAAT – which should be the first voided urine sample – and urinalysis and MSU (midstream Urine) if there are urinary symptoms, to exclude a urine tract infection.

Blood tests for HIV, syphilis and hepatitis should be done if required. If a man has an ulcer in the genital area this could be genital herpes and a swab should be taken; it could also be syphilis, so serology is important to exclude that possibility.

TYPES OF SEXUALLY TRANSMITTED INFECTIONS

Gonorrhoea

Niesseria gonorrhoea is caused by gram negative diplococcus. It may be found in the urethra, endocervix, rectum, oropharynx and conjunctiva. In asymptomatic men and women, where a NAAT test for gonorrhoea and chlamydia has been found to be positive, a culture for gonorrhoea sensitivities needs to be performed to ensure the correct treatment is given. Men who are symptomatic with gonorrhoea have a muco-purulent urethral discharge which can be very profuse. They may also have dysuria as well as pain in and swelling of their testicles. Symptomatic women may present with discharge and abdominal pain. Pharyngeal infection is asymptomatic in 90 per cent of men and women. Rectal infection is usually asymptomatic but may cause pain and discharge. This highlights why it is important to ask about the type of sexual intercourse clients have so that you can screen the relevant area.

Treatment: first line treatment, if the client is not allergic to penicillin, is Ceftriaxone 500mg given intramuscularly plus a stat dose orally of Azithromycin 1g. Clients should be advised that if they vomit within two hours they will need to repeat the dose. All sexual partners for the past three months will need to be contacted for screening and treatment. Clients should be advised to have no sexual intercourse for one week: they should return for a test of the cure in two weeks.

Chlamydia

Chlamydia is a common infection which is usually asymptomatic. Complications include pelvic inflammatory disease, ectopic pregnancy, infertility caused by fallopian tube damage in women and, in men, it can cause prostatitis and epididymoorchitis. Women may complain of dysuria, post-coital bleeding, irregular bleeding, deep dyspareunia and abdominal pain. Men may complain of clear urethral discharge, urethral irritation and dysuria. Pharyngeal infection is usually asymptomatic and rectal infection can also be asymptomatic but may also cause pain and discharge. Diagnosis is from a gonorrhoea and chlamydia NAAT swab but also, if microscopy is available, when five or more pus cells are seen on a dry slide.

Treatment: first line treatment is Azithromycin 1g orally stat and clients should be advised that if they vomit within two hours they will need to repeat the dose. The client should have no sexual intercourse for one week, and all sexual partners for the last three months should be contacted.

Trichomoniasis

Trichomonas vaginalis is found in the urethra and paraurethral glands and vagina. It is caused by a flagellated protozoan and is sexually transmitted. It is sometimes asymptomatic in men and women, but can cause increased yellow frothy vaginal discharge, itching and dysuria in women and, in men, urethral discharge and dysuria. Diagnosis is with a wet slide and microscopy, or by specialist culture testing but this is not widely available. Microscopy screening is more accurate for women and can be 80 per cent sensitive, but it is difficult to diagnose in men and can have only a 30 per cent sensitivity.

Treatment: first line treatment is Metronidazole 400mg twice daily for five days. Clients should be advised to not have sexual intercourse for one week after treatment has been completed, and all sexual contacts for the previous three months should be treated.

Syphilis

Syphilis is caused by the bacteria Treponema pallidum and can be transmitted horizontally through sexual or blood-borne infection or vertically through the placenta as congenital syphilis. It is classified into the following:

■ Early syphilis is defined as the first two years of infection.

1 *Primary*: this is syphilis within the first 90 days of infection. It is associated with a painless primary lesion known as a chancre that looks like an ulcer. The ulcer is oval or round and has a clearly defined outline.
2 *Secondary*: syphilis at 6 to 12 weeks from infection is often associated with a symmetrical rash which may be found on the trunk, limbs, face, palms of the hands and soles of the feet.

■ Early latent is defined as infection less than two years old and asymptomatic.
■ Late latent is defined as infection more than two years old and asymptomatic.
■ Tertiary or symptomatic late syphilis is untreated syphilis which can involve the musculo-skeletal, neurological and cardiovascular systems. It can result in aortic aneurysm, aortic regurgitation, paralysis, memory loss and antisocial behaviour and gumma formation (syphilitic granulation tissue).

Treatment: first line treatment is Benzathine Penicillin 2.4MU given intramuscularly in two doses a week apart in early syphilis; in late syphilis three doses are given weekly over three weeks. Clients with late syphilis should be examined to exclude any cardiac or neurological involvement. All men and women with syphilis should be advised not to have sexual intercourse until it is confirmed that they are not infectious. In early syphilis all sexual partners over the past three months will need to be traced; if it is secondary or early latent syphilis, sexual contacts for the last two years will need to be informed. Clients will require regular serology to ensure that they have been successfully treated and there is no relapse.

Genital warts

Genital warts are mostly benign and are caused by the human papillomavirus types 6 and 11. Men and women find them embarrassing and distressing. They are diagnosed through visual inspection.

Treatment: treatment for external genital warts is through cryotherapy followed by Podophyllotoxin solution 0.5 per cent treatment (if the warts are easily accessible for the client to apply treatment themselves) a week later. This is applied twice a day for three days per week for four weeks. Treatment should only be applied to broken skin and warts should be reviewed after fve weeks. Podophyllotoxin is contra-indicated in pregnancy. Warts on the cervix will need referral to colposcopy. Treatment can cause scarring and men and women should be advised to use condoms.

Genital herpes

Genital herpes is caused by the herpes simplex virus (HSV) types 1 and 2. HSV type 1 is associated with oro-labial mucosa and HSV type 2 is associated with sexually transmitted genital herpes. Men and women may complain of ulceration in the genital area; this would have started as a blister and been itchy or stinging. Depending on the location of the ulcer, it may cause problems with passing urine and may cause retention of micturition and phimosis in men. Clients may have felt generally unwell and tired beforehand. Diagnosis is through a HSV swab taken from the ulcer.

Treatment: the treatment is Aciclovir 200mg orally five times a day for five days. The use of condoms is important to reduce transmission. Genital herpes has no permanent cure; clients may never get another episode or may get frequent episodes. Clients can be very distressed; they can feel betrayed that a partner has not told them of an infection and find it difficult to discuss their diagnosis with partners.

NON-SEXUALLY TRANSMITTED INFECTIONS

Bacterial vaginosis

Bacterial vaginosis (BV) is not a sexually transmitted infection and is caused by an overgrowth of anaerobic organisms in the vagina. It causes a fishy-smelling vaginal discharge, with soreness and itching. It is associated in pregnancy with premature rupture of membranes, pre-term birth and post-partum endometritis.

Treatment: first line treatment is Methronidazole 400mg twice daily for five days and contact screening is not required. If a woman suffers from recurrent BV, you may wish to refer her to a specialist clinic as she may have Trichomonas and her partner should also be treated. Women should be encouraged to avoid washing the vagina with bath and beauty products. The vagina is a self-cleaning organ and these products destroy the natural flora in the vagina, causing an overgrowth of anaerobic organisms and BV. Woman often wash more often after sexual intercourse so you will need to discuss how BV is caused to reduce recurrences.

Candida

Candida is caused by Candida albicans and is not sexually transmitted. It causes vulval itching and soreness, and discharge is white and thick like cottage cheese. Diagnosis is through a vaginal swab for microbiology or through microscopy.

Treatment: first line treatment is Clotrimazole 500mg pessary per vagina, or Fluconazole 150mg may be given orally if the woman is not pregnant. It is good practice to perform urinalysis to exclude diabetes mellitus and a full STI screen. You should also warn your client that treatment for candida may cause condoms to break.

SELF-ASSESSMENT QUESTIONS

Answers and discussion at the end of the chapter.

1. You are giving Azithromycin for chlamydial infection; what other advice do you need to give?
2. When should you perform a test of cure with gonorrhoea infection?
3. Why is it better to know you are HIV positive?

CASE STUDY 4.1

A 32-year-old woman attends and wants to be screened for sexually transmitted infections. She is asymptomatic and always uses condoms for vaginal sex. She has had three partners during the past three months, and has had oral and vaginal sex. She never uses condoms for oral sex. She performs a NAAT self-swab for chlamydia and gonorrhoea, and it is suggested that she has oral NAAT swabs for chlamydia and gonorrhoea and culture swabs for gonorrhoea sensitivities. She also has blood taken for HIV and STS. She returns two weeks later after receiving a phone call, as she has a positive gonorrhoea result. She is quite shocked as she had no idea you could get gonorrhoea in the mouth.

SEXUALITY AND ANXIETIES

Sexually transmitted infections can cause a huge amount of anxiety in men and women. While most men and women know about HIV, they often think it won't happen to them and put themselves at risk. With increasing rates of STIs being reported it is easy to say that people are taking more risks, but actually a large proportion of this is because of increasing sensitivity of diagnostic tests, and the increasing numbers of people taking up testing. Health professionals need to discuss with men and women how to negotiate screening with their partners and condom use. We also need to be open minded about sexual practices, so that men and women are able to talk about the risks they take and we can address these risks.

Clients often do not realize the intimate nature of the questions we need to ask and can feel very embarrassed; this is one reason why you should see them on their own, as they are more likely to be honest without the presence of friends or partners.

Certain STIs, such as genital herpes and HIV, will have long-term repercussions for a person's sexual life; they may feel unclean or a danger to sexual partners. Many feel they have been foolish in trusting a partner who has not divulged an infection, and feel angry and betrayed. As a result they may require psychosexual counselling, or counselling from a health adviser to adjust to their diagnosis.

ANSWERS TO SELF-ASSESSMENT QUESTIONS

1. *You are giving Azithromycin for chlamydial infection; what other advice do you need to give?*

When you give Azithromycin for treatment of chlamydia you should advise men and women to return if they vomit within two hours of taking it. They should not have sexual intercourse for one week, and not have sexual intercourse with partners until they are screened and treated, and one week after treatment has been completed.

2. *When should you perform a test of cure with gonorrhoea infection?*

Test of cure for gonorrhoea should be performed at two weeks to ensure clients have been treated successfully.

3. *Why is it better to know you are HIV positive?*

It is a good idea to know if you are HIV positive because there is HIV 1 and HIV 2. HIV 1 is more virulent than HIV 2, HIV 2 is resistant to non-nucleoside reverse transcriptase inhibitors so if you are HIV 1 positive you will have more treatment options, and can protect yourself from contracting HIV 2. With treatment your viral load will be low which will mean you will be less infectious, and progression of the infection can be monitored.

MALE METHODS

5

■ Introduction
■ Coitus interruptus
■ Condoms
■ Male sterilization
■ Future male contraception

INTRODUCTION

The choice of contraception available to a man is limited compared with that available to a woman. Most research has been aimed at female clients because it is the woman who will become pregnant and because it is easier to stop a monthly ovulation rather than a continuous sperm process. However, with increasing education and sexual openness more men are taking a keen interest in this area, as shown by the number of men opting for sterilization. Health education councils and the media have tried to promote the use of the male condom in the prevention against sexually transmitted diseases and HIV, with limited effect; there is still the belief that 'it won't happen to me', and as long as this exists the widespread use of condoms is impeded.

COITUS INTERRUPTUS

History and introduction

Coitus interruptus is where a man withdraws his penis from the vagina before ejaculating during sexual intercourse. It is the oldest method of contraception, being referred to in the Bible (Genesis 38: verse 9) and the Koran. Coitus interruptus is widely accepted and used in Muslim and Christian communities as a method of contraception. The name coitus interruptus is rarely used by men and women – instead it is usually referred to as withdrawal, although there are many other euphemisms such as 'being careful' or 'he looks after things'. This can lead to misunderstanding during consultations if you are unaware of the euphemisms used for coitus interruptus, as these can vary in different areas. You may have to clarify with the client what they are practising as a method of contraception to enable you to help them during the consultation.

Explanation of the method

This is where the man withdraws his penis from the woman's vagina before ejaculating.

Efficacy

The efficacy of coitus interruptus is variable but with careful and consistent use it can be as high as 96 per cent effective in preventing pregnancy. However, the figure may be as low as 81 per cent with less careful and committed use (Clubb and Knight, 1996). Another reason why this method may fail is the presence of sperm in pre-ejaculate.

Disadvantages

- Low efficacy.
- No protection against HIV and other sexually transmitted infections.
- May inhibit enjoyment during sexual intercourse.

Advantages

- Easily available.
- Requires no clinic appointment.
- Acceptable to certain religions.
- No financial cost.
- Under the control of the couple.

Absolute contra-indication

- Men with erectile problems such as premature ejaculation.

Decision of choice

Many couples choose to use this method because of its accessibility. This may be because they have no other contraception available at the time of intercourse or because they feel that other choices are unsuitable. Coitus interruptus is often chosen as a method by couples for its religious acceptability. It may also be used initially in a new sexual relationship or where other methods seem unacceptable to the couple.

PROBLEMS ENCOUNTERED

- Pregnancy.
- Sexual frustration.
- Anxiety over method.

Sexuality and anxieties

You may encounter anxiety in either partner. The man may feel anxious over the responsibility placed upon him to successfully withdraw his penis before ejaculation. This may reduce his enjoyment during sexual intercourse and may lead to erectile problems. The woman may experience anxiety over her partner's ability to use withdrawal and the risk of pregnancy; as a result she may complain of loss of satisfaction during intercourse.

For many couples this may be a highly acceptable form of contraception which is under their influence and easily reversible. They have the power to revoke their decision and have 'unprotected' sexual intercourse if they wish to conceive at any time.

CONDOMS

History and introduction

Condoms were one of the first forms of contraception invented. They were made from many unusual materials and were initially seen as a protection against sexually transmitted infections rather than pregnancy. Egyptian men were first reported to use condoms to protect themselves against infection back in 1350–1220 BC. Later in AD 1564 an Italian anatomist called Gabrielle Fallopius proclaimed to have invented a condom made from linen in an effort to protect against syphilis. During Casanova's era in the 1700s condoms were being used not only to protect against infection but also against pregnancy. In the past, condoms have been made from animal bladders, oiled silk, paper and leather (Durex 1993).

With the discovery of the acquired immune deficiency syndrome (AIDS) in 1981 (Conor and Kingman, 1988), condoms have been widely advertised and promoted. They may be bought in supermarkets, petrol stations and vending machines, and are available in public male and female toilets.

Condoms are a highly effective method and one of the few contraceptives available to a man. They are often referred to under a variety of names such as sheath, johnny, rubber and french letter.

Explanation of method

A condom is made from a latex sheath which is applied and covers the length of an erect penis. It is disposable and should only be used once, and comes with different features and in a variety of colours. A condom acts as a barrier preventing sperm and ovum from meeting and pregnancy occurring. Latex-free condoms or polyurethane condoms are available for clients with latex allergies.

Efficacy

The efficacy of the condom is variable – with careful and consistent use it can be as high as 98 per cent or as low as 85 per cent. The lower efficacy is more likely to occur in men and women who are younger and more fertile with less experience in using this method (Trussell *et al.*, 1994).

Disadvantages

- Perceived as messy.
- Perceived as interrupting sexual intercourse.
- Requires forward planning.
- Loss of sensitivity.
- Latex condoms cannot be used in conjunction with oil-based lubricants.
- Erectile problems: client may find applying condoms difficult.

Advantages

- Under the control of the couple.
- No systemic effects.
- Easily available.
- Protection against sexually transmitted infections and HIV.
- May protect against cervical neoplasia.

UKMEC 3 risks outweigh the benefits of using method: relative contra-indication

- Allergy to latex proteins.

Range of condoms

Condoms now come in a variety of colours, flavours and shapes. Condoms must conform to the European condom standard and bear the European CE mark. In the UK many condoms have met the British Standards Institution specification (ISO 4074). Condoms will carry the BSI Kitemark and the European Standard logo to demonstrate they have met these requirements. The use of the BSI kitemark shows that a condom complies with a recognized standard of quality and reliability. Colours available include gold, transparent, black, red, blue, coral, yellow, orange and green. Flavours include mint flavoured, strawberry, blueberry, banana and tangerine. Shapes include contoured, flared, plain-ended, straight and ribbed.

Decision of choice

For many men and women condoms are a convenient and easily accessible form of contraception. They allow men to share and take the responsibility for preventing pregnancy. Condoms can increase enjoyment by giving permission to men and women to touch and explore the penis. The application of a condom can be shared by either partner, creating equality in the relationship.

For many clients, choosing this method may be a sudden spur-of-the-moment decision. It is often used initially in a sexual relationship, and these clients are usually younger. Many men and women prefer to use condoms to protect themselves against HIV; however, there is still the belief that 'it won't happen to me'. In *The Durex Report* (1994) 46 per cent of people questioned did not believe they would contract HIV and 43 per cent of men and women between the ages of 18 and 24 had had unprotected sexual intercourse in the past year (Durex, 1994). However, many women are now using a condom for practising safer sex and another method of contraception for the prevention of pregnancy, a practice known as the 'double Dutch'. However, this is still an area that requires increased awareness and promotion as seen in more recent research. In 2010 the *Face of Global Sex* report (Durex network, 2010) compared young people from 15 Eastern and Western countries and gave KAP scores for their sexual health. A low KAP score was given for lack of awareness of risk and low levels of condom use, lack of knowledge of sexual and reproductive health and low levels of confidence in negotiating condom use. Western countries were found to have high KAP scores, while Eastern countries were found to have low KAP scores. The profile of Western countries highlighted sex education from an early age. For health professionals this confirms the importance of educating clients but also how important it is to discuss negotiating condom use.

Choosing a condom these days may be fraught with indecision for clients. How do they know which one to try? What's the difference? You are in a prime position to advise about how to use condoms, and how to help your clients choose the condom most suitable for them.

There is no legal age limit requirement that restricts the sale of condoms, and this gives condoms both a wide and young user age range. Many men and women stop using condoms because of complaints of loss of sensitivity. Often change to another method is exacerbated by a user failure such as a burst condom or a condom coming off during sexual intercourse.

It is believed that one reason why men complain of loss of sensitivity with condoms is because they are too tight. Flared and contoured condoms are designed to give more space to the head of the penis, thus alleviating this problem. Contoured condoms are anatomically shaped to hug the glans, so that they are less likely to slip off while still increasing sensitivity. Ribbed condoms are straight condoms with extra bands of latex which are designed to heighten sensitivity for a woman. Straight condoms come in designs with or without a teat (the teat is to retain ejaculate). Condoms with teats such as straight, flared or contoured should be used for internal lubrication. Internal lubrication, or 'gel charging', involves putting water-soluble lubricant into the teat of the condom. As the gel liquefies around the glans, sensitivity increases; however, this has been found to be associated with an increased risk of condom slippage, and if men and woman practise this method they should be warned of this risk (FSRH, 2012b).

Condoms vary in strength. The strongest are condoms like Mates Superstrong and Durex Ultrastrong, which are thicker. They are suitable for men who experience premature ejaculation or wish for other reasons to delay ejaculation. Condom breakage rates are similar for standard and thicker condoms so there is no requirement for thicker condoms to be used for anal intercourse (FRSH, 2012b). The female condom may be used for anal intercourse if the inner ring is removed. Although male and female condoms make anal intercourse safer in prevention of sexually transmitted infections (STIs) and HIV they are not manufactured for this use. Condoms which are thinner are designed to increase sensitivity but clients need to be aware of the need to apply these carefully: examples of these are Durex Elite or Featherlite. However, breakage rates are similar for standard and thicker condoms, which highlights how important it is to teach condom application correctly.

Polyurethane condoms were designed to alleviate some of the disadvantages of latex condoms. Unlike latex condoms polyurethane condoms are not affected by fat-soluble products; they are baggier and less restrictive around the glans of the penis causing less loss of sensitivity. It was hoped that polyurethane condoms would have a lower condom breakage rate; however, in controlled clinical trials Frezieres *et al.* (1999) found that the breakage and slippage rate for polyurethane condoms was 8.5 per cent compared to 1.6 per cent for latex condoms. The research also found that men were more satisfied with the latex condom, and participants were less likely to withdraw from the study with condom-related reasons compared to those using a polyurethane condom.

It is no longer recommended that condoms contain the spermicide Nonoxynol 9, which may give increased local irritation and increase transmission of sexually transmitted infections and HIV (FFPRHC, 2007; FSRH, 2012b). If a partner complains of local irritation caused by a condom then a condom using a non-spermicidal lubricant should be used, once genito-urinary infections have been excluded.

Flavoured condoms are suitable for oral intercourse and come in a variety of flavours and colours, as already described. Condoms are available in discreet packaging aimed at different age groups.

Loss of efficacy of the condom

Various preparations affect the efficacy of the condom. Oil-based preparations should not be used with latex-containing condoms as they damage the latex rubber. These include lipstick, body oils, massage oils, baby oils, butter, ice cream, Vaseline, etc. Vaginal and topical preparations should not be used with latex as they may cause damage; these include econasole, miconazole, isoconazole, fenticonazole and clotrimazole.

Teaching clients how to use a condom

Teaching clients how to use and apply a condom requires little time, yet may prevent user failure. Research indicates that condom breakages are more common in young and inexperienced clients (Sparrow and Lavill, 1994). Other condom failures occur where the condom has slipped off inside the vagina following loss of erection after sexual intercourse. Condom mishaps are most likely to occur at the beginning of a relationship (UK Family Planning Research Network, 1993) and decrease as the relationship continues. This means that new and transient relationships are most at risk of unprotected sexual intercourse.

All this information shows how important it is to teach clients how to use condoms. When teaching your clients it is helpful to show how to apply a condom using a condom demonstrator. Encourage your client to check that the date on the condom packet has not expired and has the BSI kitemark and CE logo. When opening the condom packet clients should push the condom out of the way to avoid tearing; the condom packet should then be squeezed, allowing the condom to slip out. A condom should be applied before the penis comes into contact with the vulva. The condom should be placed on the erect penis and unrolled carefully along the whole length of it. Using their other hand the client should squeeze the

If you are uncertain how to put on a condom, simply follow this step-by-step guide:

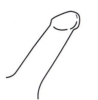

1. Put the condom on when the penis is erect, before there is any contact between the penis and your partner's body. Fluid released from the penis during the early stages of an erection can contain sperm and micro-organisms that can cause STIs.

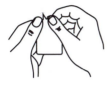

2. Tear along one side of the foil being sure not to rip the condom inside. Carefully remove the condom.

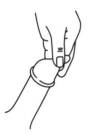

3. Air trapped inside the condom can cause it to break. To avoid this, squeeze the closed end of the condom between your forefinger and thumb and place the condom over the erect penis. Be sure the roll is on the outside.

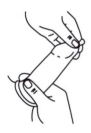

4. While still squeezing the closed end, use your other hand to unroll the condom gently down the full length of the penis. Make sure the condom stays in place during sex; if it rolls up, roll it back into place immediately. If the condom comes off, withdraw the penis and put on a new condom before intercourse continues.

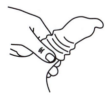

5. Soon after ejaculation, withdraw the penis while it is still erect by holding the condom firmly in place. Remove the condom only when the penis is fully withdrawn. Keep both the penis and condom clear from contact with your partner's body.

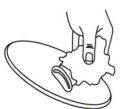

6. Never use a condom more than once – dispose of the used one hygienically, wrapping it in tissue and placing it in a bin.

Figure 5.1 How to use a condom. (Adapted from Durex SSL International plc, Cheshire)

condom at the head of the penis to expel any air. Once ejaculation has taken place the penis should be withdrawn, holding the condom on to the base of the penis to ensure that it is not left in the vagina. Condoms should only be used once (Fig. 5.1) and disposed of carefully.

You should discuss with your client the loss of efficacy caused by oil-based lubricants, and give up-to-date information on condoms. As all methods of contraception have a failure rate it is important to discuss emergency contraception. Younger women have been found to be more likely to seek emergency contraception than older women following a condom failure (UK Family Planning Research Network, 1993); this may be for a number of reasons. However, there are still large gaps in men's and women's knowledge of post-coital contraception, so this is a good time to correct misconceptions.

ACTIVITY

Practise applying condoms with either a condom demonstrator or your fingers. Do you know which condoms are available where you work?

PROBLEMS ENCOUNTERED

There are a number of accidents that can be encountered while using condoms.

The condom burst or split during sexual intercourse

This is usually because the client has either put the condom on inside-out or not released any air, or because the condom has come into contact with a fat-soluble product, (e.g. baby oil (see section on loss of efficacy on p. 50)) which has caused the condom to break.

The condom slipped off during intercourse or remained inside the vagina when the penis was withdrawn following intercourse

This usually happens when a man loses his erection and fails to hold on to the condom when he removes his penis from the vagina, leaving the condom inside the vagina. The condom can also slip off when applied inside-out.

The condom was ripped while it was being applied

This may be due to ragged nails or rings, and a new condom should be applied if this happens.

Difficulties when applying the condom: 'it's too small or too big'

Condoms can now be bought to accommodate different sizes of penis. All condoms are able to expand so it should not be too small. However, Mates now make condoms in contoured and flared shapes; flared are suitable for men who complain that the condom is too small, and contoured for men who find condoms too big. Durex also make a condom called 'Surefit' for men who want smaller sized condoms.

Allergy to condoms

Men who complain of allergy to condoms are usually allergic to the spermicide and should try a condom which does not contain a spermicide; all condoms are hypoallergenic.

Loss of sensitivity

Condoms that are plain-ended and thin will help increase sensitivity. Men may complain of loss of sensitivity because the condom is too tight; flared condoms may help alleviate this problem.

CASE STUDY 5.1

A 33-year-old married woman consulted concerned that she had a condom left inside her vagina. The condom was found and removed from the vagina. During the session the nurse asked whether emergency contraception was wanted, and whether the woman was happy with her method of contraception.

The woman was trying to conceive, but explained that the condom was from another partner and she would therefore want emergency contraception. As she had already had unprotected sexual intercourse with her regular partner with whom she was trying to conceive throughout her cycle, and was now beyond the limits for emergency contraception, this was contra-indicated. The risks of this episode of unprotected sexual intercourse were discussed in relation to pregnancy and genito-urinary infection. A pregnancy test was performed which was negative and a further test was arranged for a week's time when the client's next period was due.

SELF-ASSESSMENT QUESTIONS

Answers and discussion at the end of the chapter.

1   What sort of condom would you recommend for anal intercourse?
2   Name ten products which will cause condoms to burst.

The future

In the future any condom that is designed to minimize condom breakages or has a higher efficacy is likely to receive a warm welcome. Research has focused on different condoms and packaging; recently Ben Pawle has designed a condom cover which can be opened by the flick of a finger. This will be particularly useful for men who do not have full mobility following cardiovascular accidents, but will also be useful to all, as it may reduce breakages when opening packets.

Sexuality and anxieties

There are many different perceptions regarding the use of condoms. Studies in the USA have shown (Grady *et al.*, 1993) that many men believe that using a condom 'shows you care'; however, at the same time it may give other messages (e.g. 'that you have HIV' or 'that you think that your partner has HIV'). These anxieties cause a dilemma for men and women, and illustrate how difficult it is to talk to a new partner about sexual intercourse and safer sex. The embarrassment this causes may be the reason why so many couples have unprotected sexual intercourse.

Men and women often consult following accidents with condoms for emergency contraception. New relationships appear to be the riskiest time for condom breakages (UK Family Planning Research Network, 1993). However, research with commercial sex workers in the USA (Albert *et al.*, 1995) suggests that regular condom use leads to the development of techniques which reduce breakage and slippage of condoms. When clients consult for emergency contraception following a condom breakage this is a prime opportunity to discuss condom technique and alleviate any future problems. Many men and women use a condom breakage as their reason for requiring emergency contraception when in fact they have had unprotected sexual intercourse which they feel will be disapproved of by professionals. This makes it difficult to obtain accurate statistics for condom use and breakage.

Condoms give a man the opportunity to take part in contraception; they are often used at some point in a relationship, and have the advantage of taking care of the 'mess'. However, for some women this may be the very reason why they dislike condoms; the 'mess' or ejaculate may be warm and exciting.

Condoms can give a woman permission to touch her partner's penis; she can use a condom as part of a safe form of foreplay by applying it herself or together with her partner. This can give couples the opportunity to talk about their sexual needs and desires.

MALE STERILIZATION

History and introduction

Male sterilization has become a popular choice of permanent contraception for many couples; the surgical procedure is known as a vasectomy. The first experiments into occlusion of the vas deferens were conducted as early as 1830 by Sir Astley Cooper, and later in the twentieth century, with the advancement of surgery and anaesthesia, vasectomies became available for men. This resulted in the Family Planning Association opening its first vasectomy clinic in October 1968.

Explanation of the method

A vasectomy involves cutting the vas deferens, which is the tube that transports sperm from the epididymis in the testes to the seminal vesicles. By cutting the vas deferens, sperm is unable to be ejaculated and a man will become infertile once the vas deferens is clear of sperm, which takes about three months.

Efficacy

A vasectomy is a highly effective form of contraception. Its immediate failure rate is 1 in 2000 (RCOG, 2004).

Disadvantages

- Alternative contraception is required until two consecutive clear sperm counts are obtained.
- Surgical procedure is required.
- Local or general anaesthesia is required.
- Not easily reversible.

Advantages

- Permanent method.
- High efficacy.
- Removal of anxiety of unplanned pregnancy.
- Safe and simple procedure.

Absolute contra-indications

- Serious physical disability.
- Urological problems.
- Relationship problems.
- Indecision by either partner.

Range of method

During a vasectomy the vas deferens will be cut and either cautery or a ligature will be applied. Part of the incised vas deferens may be sent to pathology to confirm that the correct tube has been cut. Each end of the vas deferens will be buried in separate tissue layers to prevent them from rejoining (see Fig. 5.2). Research comparing traditional surgery for vasectomies with electrocautery non-scalpel vasectomy techniques found that men experienced less pain and bleeding from the wound with this method (Black, 2003). The non-scalpel method is now the recommended choice for a vasectomy surgery (RCOG, 2004).

Male sterilization (vasectomy)

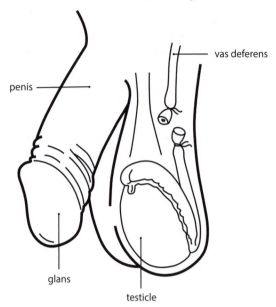

Figure 5.2 Male sterilization. (Adapted from FPA, 'Your guide to male and female sterilisation', November 2012, p. 7)

Side effects

- Infection.
- Haematoma.
- Sperm granuloma.

Counselling a couple for a vasectomy

Vasectomy counselling is preferably performed with both partners, as this is a decision which will permanently affect both parties. As this is a permanent method of contraception the couple should be sure of their decision, and aware that the procedure is very difficult to reverse. Couples during counselling are often asked to consider certain scenarios (e.g. how they would feel if their partner died, whether they would want to have more children, if they have not had children whether there is a likelihood that they will change their mind). Sometimes clients have not considered major life events and their effects, and during counselling may decide to delay such a permanent decision.

Men are often concerned about their ability to maintain erections and have sexual intercourse following a vasectomy. You can advise your clients that a vasectomy does not affect libido or erections and their ejaculate will look the same except it will no longer contain sperm, which is not detectable to the human eye.

It is important that your client continues to use an effective form of contraception, as it may cause considerable distress if a client has a vasectomy and then finds his partner is pregnant. Contraception will be required for about three months following a vasectomy. Once two consecutive negative sperm counts have been obtained then the use of another form of contraception may be ceased.

There has been concern over an increased incidence of testicular (West, 1992) and prostate cancer (Giovannucci *et al.*, 1993a, b) in men who have had a vasectomy. At the moment there is no increased link between cancer of the prostate or testes and vasectomies (RCOG, 2004). It may be that men who have had a vasectomy are more aware and consult earlier if they notice a problem (Howards and Peterson, 1993). Smoking increases the risk of all cancers, including testicular and prostate cancer. Cancer of the prostate is a disease usually found in older men; 90 per cent of all deaths from cancer of the prostate occur after the age of 65.

Vasectomies can fail even after negative sperm counts and it is important to discuss this with your client beforehand (Brahams, 1995). This is thought to be due to re-canalization of the vas deferens.

Procedure

A vasectomy may be performed under local or general anaesthetic. One or two incisions are made on each scrotum so that the vas deferens may be located, excised and ligated.

Post-vasectomy

Men should be encouraged to take things gently, as this will reduce the risk of bruising. They should wear a scrotal support and avoid heavy lifting, strenuous exercise and sexual intercourse for a week post-operatively. Pain may be eased by the use of ice packs and analgesia; frozen peas are suitable for this purpose as they mould around the area well, reducing swelling and pain. A follow-up study of men who had had a vasectomy (Canter and Goldthorpe, 1995) found that the median time to full recovery after the operation was seven days. Many clients do not allow enough time for full recovery, which increases their chances of getting post-operative complications.

Once a man has had two consecutive sperm tests which are clear of sperm then he can stop using another form of contraception. It takes about three months for a man's ejaculate to clear of sperm.

Following a vasectomy a man should watch for any signs of infection, haematoma and sperm granuloma. Any signs of rising temperature and/or pain or swelling around the testes may indicate infection, which will need to be treated with antibiotics. A haematoma is likely to occur if a client has not given himself enough time to recuperate; it should be treated with ice packs, analgesia and rest. A sperm granuloma can cause pain and localized swelling but can also be asymptomatic; it occurs when sperm leaks into the surrounding tissue where the vas deferens was excised and may need further excision.

Reversal of vasectomy

Reversal is often requested when a man has commenced a new relationship and wishes to have children. Reversal of a vasectomy is easier to perform than reversal of a female sterilization. However, success is variable and can be between 52 to 82 per cent successful in achieving a pregnancy (RCOG, 2004); this may be higher in skilled hands and may be lower if the operation was performed more than ten years ago. When reversing a vasectomy the vas deferens is re-anastomosed, which may be successful, but there is a risk that anti-sperm antibodies will develop and cause the sperm count to be low, making pregnancy difficult to achieve.

SELF-ASSESSMENT QUESTIONS

Answers and discussion at the end of the chapter.

3   Roughly how long does it take for a man to achieve a negative sperm count following a vasectomy?
4   What advantages do you think a vasectomy has over female sterilization?
5   What anxieties may a man have over a vasectomy?

ACTIVITY

Do you know what facilities are available locally for men requesting a vasectomy? Is there a waiting list? What are your clients told about aftercare? Are you all giving out the same information?

Sexuality and anxieties

Vasectomies have become more fashionable in recent times, and this coincides with the 'sharing, caring image' of 'new men'. However, sometimes it can be used as an emotional weapon – women may say 'it's his turn to do something now', which may cause conflict in the future in their relationship. There can be an element of self-sacrifice and martyrdom about the decision, which is why meeting both parties at the counselling session may help to bring this into the open for discussion.

A vasectomy may be chosen following completion of a family but also may be the result of an unplanned pregnancy, which may scare a couple into making a decision.

Following a vasectomy some men may experience signs of grief over their loss of fertility and sexuality. This will depend on how the man feels about his decision; if he feels forced or coerced into the decision then he may feel anger and sadness over his loss. Some men see a vasectomy as tantamount to castration, and have anxieties that their ability to function as a man will be impaired permanently. Many men see a vasectomy as their opportunity to do something, especially after their partner has had children. This can cement their relationship and bring them closer, reducing anxiety over further pregnancy.

FUTURE MALE CONTRACEPTION

Research is currently being undertaken into male hormonal contraception containing testosterone and progestogen. Weekly injections of testosterone enanthate 200mg have been shown to produce azoospermia in about two-thirds of men within three months and serve oligospermia in the remaining men (Bonn, 1996). However, trials are being commenced on testosterone bucyclate which offers the advantage of longer-term contraception requiring one injection every three to four months. Sperm production can be suppressed by progestogen but testosterone is required to maintain steady drug levels in the blood and maintain suppression.

Some women feel that men cannot be relied upon to be responsible for using a hormonal method as they do not have to suffer the long-term effects of pregnancy. However, today men are increasingly interested in and prepared to accept the responsibility of sharing contraception.

ANSWERS TO SELF-ASSESSMENT QUESTIONS

1   *What sort of condom would you recommend for anal intercourse?*

As condoms are not manufactured for anal intercourse there are no recommendations for the type of condom to use for anal intercourse. Condom breakage rates are similar for standard and thicker condoms. A water-based lubricant should be used in conjunction with a condom for anal intercourse to reduce breakages.

2   *Name ten products which will cause condoms to burst.*

Oil-based preparations should not be used with latex-containing condoms as they damage the latex rubber; these include lipstick, body oils, massage oils, baby oils, butter, ice cream, Vaseline, etc. Vaginal and topical preparation should not be used with latex as they may cause damage; these include econasole, miconazole, isoconazole, fenticonazole and clotrimazole.

3   *Roughly how long does it take for a man to achieve a negative sperm count following a vasectomy?*

It takes roughly three months for a man to achieve a negative sperm count, and he can consider it safe to have sexual intercourse when he has had two consecutive negative sperm counts.

4   *What advantages do you think a vasectomy has over female sterilization?*

A vasectomy can easily be performed under local anaesthetic, while the majority of female sterilizations are performed under general anaesthetic. Anatomically, the scrotum and vas deferens are easy to locate, while with a woman, locating the fallopian tubes is harder as they are positioned under muscle and fat layers. This is why women may be in hospital for longer while a man may go home following the procedure.

5   *What anxieties may a man have over a vasectomy?*

Men have anxieties over their ability to achieve an orgasm, maintain an erection and changes in their ejaculate. Most of their anxieties surround myths about vasectomy which include impotence and sexual dysfunction. They may also have anxieties over prostate and testicular cancer. Some men may have anxieties about the procedure and fears about what may happen.

FEMALE BARRIER METHODS

6

- Introduction
- History
- The diaphragm
- The FemCap
- The female condom
- Spermicides

INTRODUCTION

Contraception not only gives women protection against pregnancy, it also gives women power over their bodies. It allows women the opportunity to choose when to conceive or not, offering them the chance to develop their lives through education and careers. However, this also creates dilemmas: by having highly effective contraception women now have to decide when to conceive, and sometimes there never seems to be a right time to do this! Many women leave trying to conceive till late into their thirties, and then find they have difficulty becoming pregnant; other women have contraceptive failures which may subconsciously stem from their desire to become pregnant.

HISTORY

Contraception has changed dramatically over the past ten years with the launch of longer-term methods such as Nexplanon and Mirena. These methods give an excellent alternative to sterilization and offer a wider choice to all women. The female condom has given women the opportunity to practise safer sex; not only is it easily inserted but it is also available over the counter in chemists.

THE DIAPHRAGM

Introduction and history

Women have used a variety of materials as barrier methods in the past, such as oiled cloth, sponges, leaves and fruit often soaked in vinegar or lemon juice. A German doctor named Hasse, who used the pseudonym Mesinga, is credited with the introduction of the diaphragm in 1882 which gave women greater freedom over their bodies. It was not until 1974 that all contraception was provided free of charge to men and women. Earlier, women had to give proof of marriage, as contraception was not available to non-married women until the late 1960s. There were three types of cervical cap – the cervical, the vimule and the vault – and these were made from rubber, smaller than a diaphragm, covering the cervix only and held in place by suction.

In recent years the variety of cervical caps and spermicides has reduced so that the only cervical cap available is the FemCap, and the only spermicide is Gygel. This is a shame, since there is still a strong following by women using diaphragms and cervical caps; and it is important that health professionals maintain the skill of being able to fit diaphragms and cervical caps as there is a risk that this will become a lost skill.

Explanation of method

The diaphragm is a dome made from either rubber or silicone which is inserted into the vagina (see Fig. 6.1). It covers the cervix, acting as a barrier to sperm and therefore helping to prevent pregnancy.

Efficacy

With careful and consistent use the diaphragm, when used with a spermicide, is 92 to 96 per cent effective in preventing pregnancy in the first year. With typical use, where a woman does not use this method, with spermicide, carefully, it is 82 to 90 per cent effective in preventing pregnancy in the first year (Bounds, 1994). Failure rates for the diaphragm depend on how effectively the woman uses it. Does she use the diaphragm for every episode of sexual intercourse? Is her cervix covered each episode? Is she using her diaphragm according to guidelines? Other factors which influence the failure rate of all methods are a woman's age and how often she is having sexual intercourse. For example, if a woman is aged 40 and uses a diaphragm as a contraceptive she is less fertile than a woman aged 25, so a diaphragm is a more effective contraceptive for her.

The use of a spermicide with the diaphragm is currently recommended. The only study which compared the diaphragm with and without spermicide (Bounds et al., 1995) did not give significant results for the use of a diaphragm being effective if used alone. Until research proves that a diaphragm is as effective without spermicide as it is with spermicide, current guidelines recommend that you teach your client to continue to use the diaphragm with a spermicide.

Disadvantages

- Requires motivation.
- Needs to be used carefully and consistently for optimum efficacy.
- Needs to be used with a spermicide which may be perceived as messy.
- May increase the risk of cystitis and urinary tract infections.
- No protection against HIV.

Advantages

- Under the control of the woman.
- May give some protection against cervical cancer and sexually transmitted diseases.
- No systemic side effects.
- Provides vaginal lubrication.
- May be used during menstruation.
- Gives a woman permission to touch and explore her body.

UKMEC 3 risks outweigh the benefits of using method: relative contra-indication

- Allergy to rubber or spermicide.
- Pregnancy.
- Undiagnosed genital tract bleeding should be investigated and treated first.
- Poor vaginal muscle tone or prolapse.
- Congenital abnormality such as two cervices or septal wall defects (where the vagina is separated into two by a wall).
- Present vaginal, cervical or pelvic infection should be investigated and treated first.
- Past history of toxic shock syndrome.
- HIV – use of spermicides containing Nonoxynol 9 is associated with genital lesions and may increase the risk of acquiring HIV or other infections.

UKMEC 2, A condition where the advantages of using the method generally outweigh the risks

- Women who feel unable to touch their genital area because of personal or religious reasons.
- Recurrent urinary tract infections.

Side effects

- Urinary tract infection.
- Toxic shock syndrome – associated with diaphragms being worn for more than 30 hours.
- Vaginal irritation.

Range of method

There are three main types of diaphragm.

The flat spring diaphragm

This type of diaphragm has a flat spring in the rim of the diaphragm, is available in sizes 55 to 95mm (rising in steps of 5mm) and is made from rubber. It is suitable for women with an anterior or mid-plane positioned cervix.

Coiled spring diaphragm

This type of diaphragm has a coiled spring in the rim of the diaphragm, is available in sizes 55 to 95mm (rising in steps of 5mm) and is made from silicone. This type of diaphragm is suitable for women who find a flat spring diaphragm uncomfortable either because they have strong vaginal muscles or they are sensitive to vaginal pressure. It is also recommended for women with a shallow symphysis pubis.

Arcing spring diaphragm

This type of diaphragm is available in sizes 55 to 95mm (rising in steps of 5mm) and is made from silicone. This type of diaphragm is suitable for women with a posterior positioned cervix, or where a woman has difficulty feeling her cervix.

Decision of choice

The decision of the type of diaphragm you fit your client with will depend on a vaginal examination. You will need to assess the vagina and cervix to exclude infection, poor muscle tone and prolapse. To estimate the size of diaphragm required, when examining your client you should measure the distance from the posterior fornix (the area immediately behind the cervix) to the symphysis pubis (the bone in front of the bladder) with your fingers (Fig. 6.1). The measurement

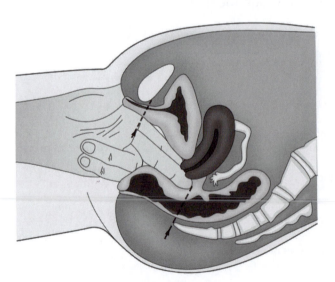

Figure 6.1 Estimating the size of the diaphragm to be fitted. (Adapted from *Handbook of Family Planning*, 2nd edn, N. Loudon (ed.), 1991, Churchill Livingstone)

on your fingers corresponds to the size of diaphragm required for your client (Fig. 6.2). With practice you will find that this is not difficult; it can be useful beforehand to see where a diaphragm measures on your fingers. The diaphragm should be fitted now to check that the correct size has been chosen (Figs 6.3 and 6.4). The diaphragm should cover the cervix and sit tucked up behind the symphysis pubis. If it protrudes into the introitus then the diaphragm is either too large (Fig. 6.5)

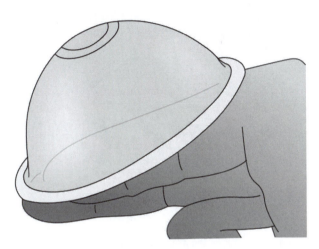

Figure 6.2 Size of diaphragm on hand. (Adapted from *Handbook of Family Planning*, 2nd edn, N. Loudon (ed.), 1991, Churchill Livingstone)

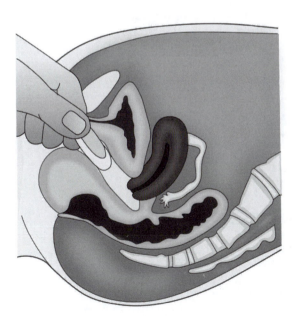

Figure 6.3 Diaphragm being inserted. (Adapted from *Handbook of Family Planning*, 2nd edn, N. Loudon (ed.), 1991, Churchill Livingstone)'

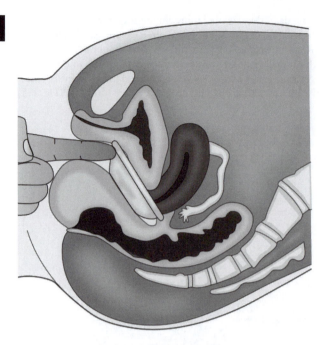

Figure 6.4 Checking the position of the diaphragm. (Adapted from *Handbook of Family Planning*, 2nd edn, N. Loudon (ed.), 1991, Churchill Livingstone)

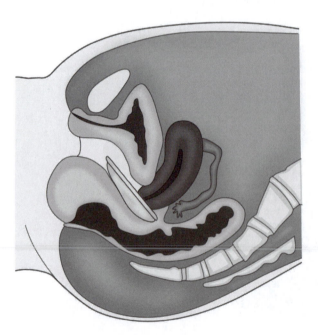

Figure 6.5 Diaphragm too large. (Adapted from *Handbook of Family Planning*, 2nd edn, N. Loudon (ed.), 1991, Churchill Livingstone)'

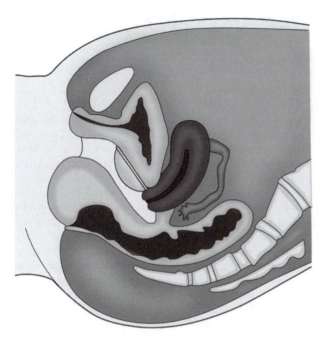

Figure 6.6 Diaphragm too small. (Adapted from *Handbook of Family Planning*, 2nd edn, N. Loudon (ed.), 1991, Churchill Livingstone)'

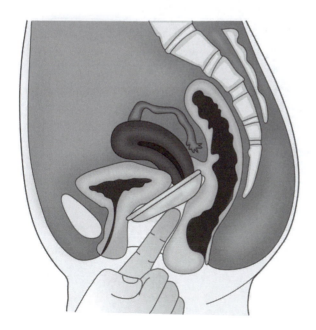

Figure 6.7 Checking a diaphragm covering the cervix (standing position). (Adapted from *Handbook of Family Planning*, 2nd edn, N. Loudon (ed.), 1991, Churchill Livingstone)'

or is fitted incorrectly. If there is a gap of a finger or more then the diaphragm is too small (Fig. 6.6). Your client should be unable to feel the diaphragm *in situ* if it is fitted correctly.

How to teach a diaphragm fitting

This can be potentially a very threatening and embarrassing situation for your client, so it is important that your examination room is quiet, private and free from interruptions. This consultation may take some time, so allow at least half an hour; you will both feel more at ease if time is not an issue. Usually a diaphragm fitting teaching session is spread over two consultations. The first visit includes initial fitting and teaching the client to locate her cervix, remove and fit the diaphragm. The second consultation includes teaching spermicidal application. Although this may be done at either visit, it is useful to have a second consultation to solve any problems. The more comfortable your client feels the more at ease she will be in the situation and the more likely she is to succeed. Before examining your client you should show her a diaphragm and, using diagrams or a teaching model, show her how the diaphragm sits inside the vagina. Some women find this slightly difficult to understand at first, and how you approach this will vary with each client. Try to find out how much she knows and build upon this. Remember that the majority of women may never have felt their cervix or thought much about its

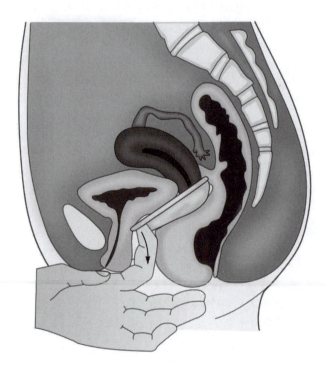

Figure 6.8 Client removing a diaphragm (standing position). (Adapted from *Handbook of Family Planning*, 2nd edn, N. Loudon (ed.), 1991, Churchill Livingstone)'

significance. Discuss how you are going to teach your client to fit her diaphragm; this will help her feel more comfortable with the situation.

Once you have estimated the correct size of diaphragm and it is *in situ*, your client should be taught to feel inside her vagina and check the position of the diaphragm and cervix. It is helpful if you wear a pair of gloves during this part of the consultation in case you need to help her by holding the diaphragm at some point. To teach your client she should be encouraged to wash her hands and either squat or put one foot on a chair. She should then feel inside her vagina so that she can understand how the diaphragm sits (Fig. 6.7). You will now need her to feel inside her vagina. It is helpful if you give your client an idea of where her cervix is positioned, and what it feels like. The cervix has been described as a fleshy lump feeling like the end of your nose. It is important that she is able to locate her cervix, so that she is aware of it being covered by the diaphragm, to ensure efficacy.

When your client is able to locate her cervix, ask her to remove her diaphragm by putting her index finger over the anterior rim of the diaphragm and pulling downwards (Fig. 6.8). The diaphragm should slip out easily. If she finds this difficult ask her to bear down, making removal easier. You may want to take the diaphragm and rinse it for your client so that it does not become too slippery initially for her to fit. She can insert the diaphragm by squeezing it together firmly with one hand, or by using her thumb and second index finger to squeeze it together while her first index finger remains inside the diaphragm, giving more control over it. The diaphragm should then be inserted into the vagina as far as it will go, pushing the anterior rim of the diaphragm underneath the ledge of the symphysis pubis. Encourage your client to check that her cervix is covered, and that she feels that the diaphragm is fitted correctly. Next check by examination that your client has fitted her diaphragm correctly.

Once your client is able to locate her cervix, fit and remove her diaphragm she is able to practise using it. Usually a second consultation is made about a week later. This allows your client time to practise, while she uses another form of contraception to avoid pregnancy. During this time she should sleep with the diaphragm *in situ*, open her bowels, have sexual intercourse, and practise removing and fitting her diaphragm, so that if she has any problems these can be discussed and solved. Occasionally it may be necessary to combine both visits into one.

At the next visit you should advise your client to come with her diaphragm already in place. By doing this you will be able to check that she is able to fit her diaphragm correctly. This is a good time to revise care of the diaphragm, how to use spermicide and how long the diaphragm should be left *in situ*. All this information should be backed up with the appropriate leaflets, details of when your client should consult early and when a routine consultation should be carried out.

You should weigh your client at both consultations, and advise her that if her weight fluctuates by 3kg either way she will need to have her diaphragm checked, and may require a smaller or larger diaphragm to be fitted.

The success of these consultations is very much down to the approach you give the session. If you are teaching your client to locate her cervix and she is having difficulty, it may be a matter of communication and confidence building. If she is using a squatting position you may find that communication between you is improved if you assume a squatting position so that you are both at the same eye level. Given time and an empathetic approach your client will gain confidence to succeed. Often clients will have problems fitting the diaphragm and locating their cervix, and may need longer at the initial consultation. Sometimes, depending on the client, you may find giving her some time by herself helpful if she feels hampered by the situation. It is important to assess each client individually; some women may require more privacy than others.

Use of the diaphragm

If your client gets into the habit of putting her diaphragm in regularly at the time she is most likely to have sexual intercourse then she is less likely to forget to put it in prior to intercourse. The diaphragm should be fitted with two 2cm strips of spermicidal gel on both sides of the diaphragm. This will give contraceptive protection for three hours. After three hours if no sexual intercourse has taken place, more spermicide will need to be inserted (e.g. a pessary). However, if sexual intercourse has taken place and further intercourse is likely later than three hours after insertion, the diaphragm should be left *in situ* and additional spermicide inserted into the vagina 5 to 10 minutes prior to intercourse to give additional cover.

The diaphragm should be left *in situ* for six hours after the last episode of sexual intercourse, but no longer than 24 hours to avoid the risk of toxic shock syndrome and pressure ulcers forming.

Finally, it is important to cover care of the diaphragm. It should be washed with mild soap and water and dried. Talcum powders, detergents and perfumes should be avoided as these will affect the natural flora in the vagina. The diaphragm should be bent back into shape and kept in its case following use. The diaphragm should be kept away from direct sunlight and radiators as these may cause the diaphragm to perish. Your client should be encouraged to check her diaphragm for holes as this will reduce its effectiveness.

Preparations that reduce the efficacy of the diaphragm

Oil-based preparations should not be used with latex-containing diaphragms as they damage the latex rubber; these include lipstick, body oils, massage oils, baby oils, butter, ice cream, Vaseline, etc. Vaginal and topical preparations should not be used with latex as they may cause damage; these include econasole, miconazole, isoconazole, fenticonazole and clotrimazole.

Subsequent visits

You should see your client routinely every six months to check that the diaphragm is being fitted correctly by her and to review her weight. The diaphragm should be renewed every year.

You should advise your client to return earlier if any of the following conditions occur:

- Her weight varies by 3kg.
- Her diaphragm deteriorates, develops a hole, etc.
- The diaphragm becomes uncomfortable.
- Pregnancy; the diaphragm should be checked following any pregnancy (e.g. miscarriage, abortion, birth).

■ She has a vaginal infection. A new diaphragm should be fitted once the infection has been investigated and treated, to prevent reinfection.

SELF-ASSESSMENT QUESTIONS

Answers and discussion at the end of the chapter.

1   Which preparations should not be used with a diaphragm?
2   How would you help a client who is unable to locate her cervix?
3   For which clients would an arcing diaphragm be appropriate?

PROBLEMS ENCOUNTERED

The following are some problems you may encounter during your consultation.

Your client is unable to locate her cervix

This may be because your client lacks confidence and needs more time. Try asking her to assume a different position, i.e. squatting or placing a foot on a chair. Sometimes you may meet a client who has regularly been using a diaphragm but has never been taught to locate her cervix.

If your client's cervix is very posterior it will be easier for her if you fit an arcing diaphragm. An arcing diaphragm has a spring which causes the diaphragm to fall naturally to the posterior part of the vagina.

The diaphragm does not cover your client's cervix

This may be because the diaphragm is too small and she needs a larger sized diaphragm or because her cervix is posterior and an arcing diaphragm is more suitable.

Your client is unable to remove her diaphragm

Ask your client to bear down, as this usually helps with removal. Remind her that the diaphragm cannot get lost. If she cannot remove it at that time she should not panic but leave removal until she is more relaxed.

Your client complains that her partner can feel the diaphragm

If your client complains that her partner can feel the diaphragm check that the diaphragm is the correct size and she is fitting it correctly.

> ## Your client complains of recurrent cystitis
>
> If your client complains of recurrent cystitis, encourage her to empty her bladder before having sexual intercourse. You should also check her diaphragm – it may be the incorrect size. If she has a flat spring diaphragm then changing her diaphragm to a coiled spring, which is softer, will help. Research has shown that women using a diaphragm were two to three times more likely to be referred with a urinary tract infection than women not using a diaphragm (Vessey, 1988), so women experiencing recurrent urine tract infections may need to review their method of contraception.

THE FEMCAP

The FemCap is the only cervical cap licensed in the UK. It is designed to conform to the natural shape of the cervix, and the brim around it serves to create a seal around the vaginal wall, preventing sperm from entering the vagina. It is made from medical grade silicone rubber and has a strap to aid removal, and may be left *in situ* for 48 hours. The FemCap should be left *in situ* for 8 hours after sexual intercourse. There are three sizes: the smallest at 22mm is intended for nulliparous women, the 26mm size is suitable for women who have been pregnant but not had a vaginal delivery, and the largest size is 30mm, suitable for women who have had a vaginal delivery. Research has found the FemCap to be 86.5 per cent effective in preventing pregnancy and, if used carefully and consistently, it may be 98 per cent effective in preventing pregnancy; what is certain is that the efficacy is no worse than the diaphragm (American Health Consultants, 2000).

Sexuality and anxieties

A client who chooses to use a diaphragm and is successful with it can find that the diaphragm gives her permission to investigate her vagina, allowing her to touch areas that may have seemed forbidden. Often women have little or no knowledge of this area of their body and have built up their own ideas about their vagina. Not only can a diaphragm act as a contraceptive, it can educate and illuminate a hidden area.

You may find that your client complains that her diaphragm is 'messy'. This may be due to real problems with a type of spermicide but often there is an underlying problem. A client who complains that her diaphragm is messy may feel that sexual intercourse is messy. Some women have fantasies about their vagina – they feel that it is a clean, sterile area and forget that it produces its own natural discharge. They find sperm messy and as a result of these feelings there may be a problem with sexual intercourse. Given time and awareness of the feelings that the client is transferring you may find that she talks about her anxieties. However, sometimes clients are not ready or able to look at their feelings, but may do so in the future.

Clients may panic if they are unable to remove their diaphragm. Behind this may lie the image that the diaphragm has disappeared into the midst of nowhere.

Through lack of knowledge men and women can create very strong images of their bodies which can be frightening and strange.

A woman who chooses the diaphragm may do so because of its lower efficacy compared to other methods. She may have a subconscious desire to become pregnant or may actively use the method to become pregnant without letting her partner know.

THE FEMALE CONDOM

Introduction and history

Women have inserted a wide variety of objects into their vaginas, from lemons to oiled silk, in order to control their fertility. The female condom is available over the counter to all women and has helped to increase the choice open to them.

Explanation of the method

The female condom is made from lubricated polyurethane. It is 170mm in length and has an outer ring and an inner ring. The inner ring, which is situated at the closed end of the condom, is used to aid insertion. The outer ring is situated at the open end of the condom and lies flat against the vulva. The female condom prevents sperm from entering the vagina by acting as a barrier.

Efficacy

The female condom is similar to the male condom in its effectiveness in preventing pregnancy. There have only been a few studies researching the efficacy of the female condom, but these indicate that the efficacy is similar to that of the male condom – from 85 per cent for typical use to 98 per cent for perfect use (Trussell *et al.*, 1994).

Disadvantages

- Perceived as noisy.
- Requires motivation.
- May be perceived as interrupting sexual intercourse.

Advantages

- Under the control of the woman.
- Protects against sexually transmitted infections and HIV.
- May be used in conjunction with oil-based products.
- No systemic side effects.

Range of method

There is one female condom available in the UK.

How to teach the use of the female condom

You should advise your client to insert the female condom by squeezing the smaller ring at the closed end of the condom between her thumb and index finger. She should then insert the ring into the vagina as far as she can and insert her finger into the condom. This will push the condom upward into the vagina, and allow the outer ring to lie flat against the vulva. The inner ring does not need to lie over the cervix, and should be left *in situ* (see Fig. 6.9).

The woman's partner should insert his penis into the condom, with the outer ring lying flat against the vulva. Care should be taken that the penis is not inserted between the condom and the vagina. Once ejaculation has taken place the outer ring should be twisted so that the ejaculate is retained in the female condom, and gently pulled out of the vagina. The female condom should be disposed of in a rubbish bin; it cannot be flushed down a toilet.

1   The small ring which lies within the closed end of the condom helps to insert the female condom much like a tampon and holds the condom in place in the vagina. To insert, firmly hold the small ring between the thumb and middle finger.

2   Find a comfortable position; either lie down, sit with the knees apart, or stand with one foot up on a chair. Insert the squeezed ring into the vagina, pushing it inside as far as possible.

3   Insert a finger inside the condom and push the small ring inside as far as it will go, like a tampon. Most women do not feel the inner ring once the female condom is inserted. Some may find that insertion is fully completed by the penis when it enters the vagina. There is no need for the female condom to be fitted over the cervix.

4   It is normal for part of the condom to hang outside the body. The outer ring helps keep the condom in place and will lie flat against the body when the penis is inside the condom. Most couples do not feel the outer ring during use.

5   The penis should be guided inside the condom. As long as the penis remains inside the sheath and the outer ring remains outside the body, then the female condom is working.

6   To remove the female condom, twist the outer ring to contain the semen and gently pull the condom out. The female condom must be removed before risk of spilling any ejaculate, immediately after loss of erection.

Like male condoms, female condoms can only be used once and must not be flushed down the toilet.

All teaching should be supported by relevant written information.

The female condom is suitable for women with a latex allergy. It is also ideal for women who are concerned about HIV and sexually transmitted infections. It feels stronger and more durable than a male condom and is not affected by oil-based lubricants.

Female barrier methods

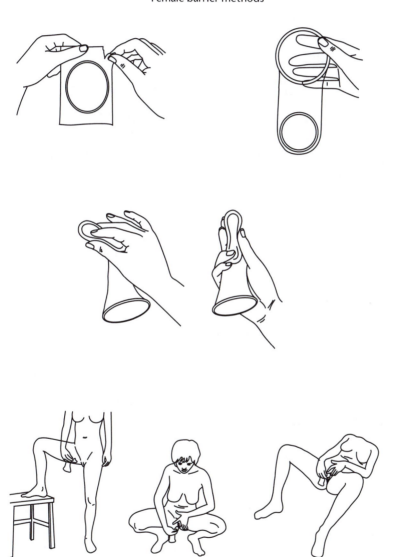

Figure 6.9 Step-by-step guide to using the female condom. (Adapted from Femidom Advice Bureau, Chartex International Plc)

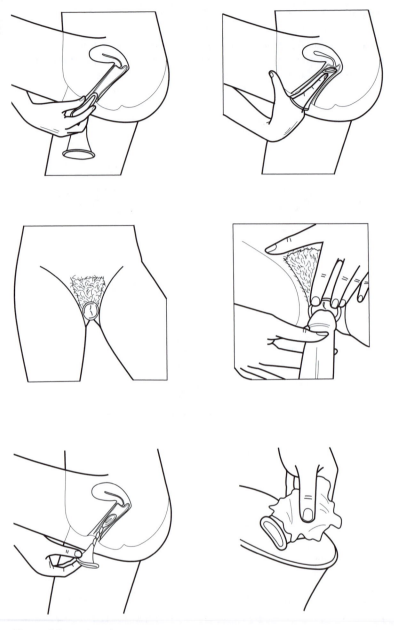

Figure 6.9 continued

Women can insert the female condom prior to sexual intercourse. They will find that it will stay *in situ* if they move around as long as they have fitted it correctly. Some women have mistakenly removed the inner ring of the condom which helps keep the condom in position.

Although research (Bounds *et al.*, 1992a) has shown that the female condom is not aesthetically pleasing to many women and their partners, a number of positive features were highlighted. These included that the Female condom rarely split, and that there was less loss of sensitivity experienced by men compared with the male condom.

PROBLEMS ENCOUNTERED

Penis inserted outside the female condom

Clients should be advised to insert the penis carefully and be aware of this problem, and informed about emergency contraception.

Female condom removed as the penis is withdrawn

Clients should be encouraged to hold onto the outside ring as the penis is withdrawn.

Client complains of noise

Some women have complained about a rustling noise when using the female condom; others, however, have commented that they do not mind the sound. The use of additional spermicide or lubrication may help to reduce this problem but this may make the condom more slippery.

SELF-ASSESSMENT QUESTIONS

Answers and discussion at the end of the chapter.

4   What advantages do you think the female condom has that would appeal to a woman?

Sexuality and anxieties

The female condom may seem unappealing to some women because of its appearance or the 'rustling sound' made when in use. However, in a relationship that is open and understanding this method may be a very acceptable choice. Research (Bounds *et al.*, 1992a) has shown that a small proportion of couples may prefer this method over the male condom, as they find sexual intercourse more enjoyable. Other couples have experienced less loss of sensitivity with the female condom.

In another study where the female condom's acceptability and experience was researched (Ford and Mathie, 1993) clients commented that they liked the 'lack of mess'. Some women encouraged their partners to insert the condom, which they found enjoyable. Other women found the insertion of the female condom embarrassing and awkward. It was also noted that, like all methods, men and women found insertion easier with prolonged use.

SPERMICIDES

Introduction and history

Spermicides are generally used with another method of contraception such as the diaphragm and condom.

Explanation of the method

Spermicides inactivate sperm by causing changes in the cell membrane of the spermatozoa.

Efficacy

There is little information about the efficacy of spermicides used on their own. They are believed to be of only a moderate efficacy, which is why it is recommended that they are used in conjunction with another form of contraception.

Disadvantages

- Perceived as messy.
- Local allergic reaction.
- Only of moderate contraceptive efficacy.

Advantages

- Provides lubrication.
- Easily available.
- May provide protection against sexually transmitted infections and HIV.
- May be used in conjunction with the barrier methods of contraception.

Absolute contra-indication

- Allergic reaction to spermicides.

Range of method

Spermicides are available in the form of Gygel.

- Local irritation.

Counselling

There is no evidence that condoms lubricated with spermicides increase efficacy, and the addition of spermicide to condoms during vaginal sex is not recommended, as it can increase condom slippage (FSRH, 2012b). Nonoxynol 9 has been demonstrated in laboratory research to be effective *in vitro* against HIV (Chantler, 1992). However, it has been found to increase the risk of genital lesions in the rectum and vagina which may increase HIV transmission. Nonoxynol 9 is therefore not recommended for use with condoms (FSRH, 2012b).

The future

Research into spermicides is currently focused on spermicides which are effective against HIV, and the dispensers that deliver them. Single-dose dispensers which can be used easily by a woman to give her protection against sexually transmitted infections and HIV prior to sexual intercourse are being considered. Research is investigating the use as a vaginal spermicide of Chlorhexidine which has shown some exciting properties. Chlorhexidine has been demonstrated to be active against HIV without the membrane disruption associated with Nonoxynol 9 (Chantler, 1992). Other areas of research have been with a new spermicide, Benzalkonium Chloride, in the formulation of a vaginal pessary, and a study on its acceptability showed less discharge and discomfort (Aubeny *et al.*, 2000).

Spermicides are seen as an extremely important area of contraception. If research can produce an acceptable spermicide for women which causes less irritation but kills HIV then it is hoped that the increased spread of HIV may be reduced.

ANSWERS TO SELF-ASSESSMENT QUESTIONS

1   *Which preparations should not be used with a diaphragm?*

The following preparations should not be used with a diaphragm, as they damage the latex rubber: lipstick, body oils, massage oils, baby oils, butter, ice cream, Vaseline. Vaginal and topical preparations should not be used with latex, as they may cause damage; these include econasole, miconazole, isoconazole, fenticonazole and clotrimazole.

2   *How would you help a client who is unable to locate her cervix?*

If a client is unable to locate her cervix, try getting her to assume a different position to feel her cervix, such as squatting or putting one foot up on a chair. You can ask if she and her partner are willing for her partner to check that her cervix is covered.

3   *For which clients would an arcing diaphragm be appropriate?*

An arcing diaphragm is suitable for a woman with a posterior cervix, or for someone who is having problems locating her cervix or fitting her diaphragm.

4   *What advantages do you think the female condom has that would appeal to a woman?*

The female condom has many advantages that appeal to women. Women who have anxiety over sexually transmitted infections and HIV because their partner has sexual intercourse outside their relationship have commented that they prefer this method because it gives them control over contraception combined with safer sex. The female condom may appeal to women who suffer from recurrences in genital herpes. It also gives a wider choice for sex workers practising safer sex.

The female condom may appeal to women who are physically disabled, as it has no systemic effects and can be inserted by her partner as part of foreplay. Any woman or her partner who has an allergy to latex may find the female condom more suitable, since it is made from polyurethane.

COMBINED METHODS

7

■ Introduction and history
■ The combined contraceptive pill
■ The combined contraceptive patch
■ The combined ring

INTRODUCTION AND HISTORY

The combined pill is today one of the most widely used methods of contraception, but the pills currently used are quite different from the original pills. In the late 1930s Dr Kurzrok showed that the administration of oral oestrogen eased dysmenorrhoea and inhibited ovulation. In 1956 clinical trials began in Puerto Rico on a combined oestrogen and progestogen pill called Enovid; it was approved for use in America in 1957. In 1960 clinical trials began in the UK and in 1961 Conovid E and Anovlar, each containing more than 50g of oestrogen, were approved by the Medical Advisory Council of the Family Planning Association.

THE COMBINED CONTRACEPTIVE PILL

Explanation of the method

The combined oral contraceptive pill contains the hormones oestrogen and progestogen. It prevents pregnancy by:

■ Inhibiting ovulation.
■ Making the endometrium unfavourable for implantation.
■ Making the cervical mucus impenetrable to sperm.

Efficacy

The efficacy for the combined pill is over 99 per cent with careful and consistent use; however, with less careful use it can be 91 per cent (FSRH, 2011a).

Disadvantages

- Needs to be taken regularly, carefully and consistently.
- No protection against STIs and HIV.
- Increased risk of circulatory disorders such as hypertension, arterial disease and venous thromboembolism.
- Increased risk of liver adenoma, cholestatic jaundice and gallstones.
- Effect of COC on breast cancer (see p. 92).
- Unsuitable for smokers over the age of 35.

Advantages

- Reliable and easily reversible.
- Relief of dysmenorrhoea and menorrhagia.
- Reduces risk of anaemia.
- Reduces the risk of benign breast disease.
- Relief of premenstrual symptoms.
- Fewer ectopic pregnancies.
- Reduction of ovarian cysts.
- Less pelvic inflammatory disease.
- Protects against endometrial and ovarian cancer.

UKMEC 4 unacceptable health risk: absolute contra-indication

- Pregnancy.
- Breast-feeding.
- Less than six weeks post-partum.
- Undiagnosed vaginal or uterine bleeding.
- Past or present venous thrombosis.
- Past or present arterial thrombosis.
- Cardiovascular and ischaemic heart disease.
- Complicated pulmonary hypertension, atrial fibrillation and subacute bacterial endocarditis.
- Migraine with aura.
- Cerebrovascular accident and transient ischaemic attacks.
- Active disease of the liver (e.g. malignancy, history of cholestatic jaundice, impaired liver function tests, acute viral hepatitis, severe cirrhosis).
- Current breast cancer.
- Systemic lupus erythematosus with positive antiphospholipid antibodies.
- Raynaud's disease with lupus anticoagulant; if present this will increase coagulation.
- Stevens–Johnson syndrome.
- Acute pancreatitis.
- Four weeks before major surgery or leg surgery.
- Known thrombogenic mutations such as Factor V Leiden, Prothrombin mutation, Protein S and Protein C and Antithrombin deficiencies.
- Severe diabetes mellitus with complications such as retinopathy, neuropathy, vascular disease.

■ Smokers over the age of 35.
■ Hypertension with a diastolic over 95mm Hg.

UKMEC 3 risks outweigh the benefits of using method: relative contra-indication

■ Obesity (body mass index (BMI) over 35kg m^{-2}).
■ Lipid disorders and diseases where high-density lipoprotein (HDL) is reduced (e.g. diabetes, hypertension).
■ Migraine without aura.
■ Past history of migraine with aura at any age.
■ Carriers of known gene mutations linked to breast cancer BRCAS 1.
■ Past history of breast cancer in the last five years.
■ History of cholestasis with a combined method.
■ Gallstones.
■ Diseases whose drug treatment affects the efficacy of the combined pill (e.g. tuberculosis, epilepsy).
■ Family history of arterial or venous disease in a first-degree relative below the age of 45.

Range of method

Drug manufacturers have produced a wide range of combined pills (Table 7.1). There are three types of combined pills:

1 Monophasic pills.
2 Biphasic pills.
3 Triphasic pills.

Monophasic pills

The most widely used combined pill is a monophasic pill, which means that it contains the same amount of oestrogen and progestogen throughout its 21-day course (e.g. Brevinor, Cilest, Eugynon 30, Femodene, Femodette, Gederal 30/150, Katya 30/75, Levest, Loestrin 20, Loestrin 30, Marvelon, Mercilon, Microgynon, Millinette 20/75, Millinette 30/75, Minulet, Ovranette, Ovysmen, Ovran, Ovran 30, Norinyl-1, Norimin, Rigevidon, Sunya 20/75, Yasmin).

There are six 20 microgram pills: Mercilon, Gederal 20/150, Femodette, Loestrin 20, Millinette 20/75, Sunya 20/75.

Biphasic pills

These follow a 21-day course and contain the same amount of oestrogen throughout the packet but have pills containing two different levels of progestogen. These are usually coded in different colours (e.g. Binovum).

Table 7.1 Combined contraceptive pills

Combined pill name	Preparation	Manufacturer	Micrograms of oestrogen per pill	Micrograms of progestogen per pill	Type of progestogen
Gedarel 150/20	21-day monophasic pill	Consilient	20mcg	150mcg	Desogestrel
Mercilon	21-day monophasic pill	Organon	20mcg	150mcg	Desogestrel
Femodette	21-day monophasic pill	Bayer Schering	20mcg	75mcg	Gestodene
Millinette 20/75	21-day monophasic pill	Consilient	20mcg	75mcg	Gestodene
Sunya	21-day monophasic pill	Stragen	20mcg	75mcg	Gestodene
Loestrin 20	21-day monophasic pill	Galen	20mcg	1mg	Northisterone acetate
Gedarel	21-day monophasic pill	Consilient	30mcg	150mcg	Desogestrel
Marvelon	21-day monophasic pill	Organon	30mcg	150mcg	Desogestrel
Yasmin	21-day monophasic pill	Bayer Schering	30mcg	3mg	Drospirenone
Femodene	21-day monophasic pill	Bayer Schering	30mcg	75mcg	Gestodene
katya	21-day monophasic pill	Stragen	30mcg	75mcg	Gestodene
Millinette 30/175	21-day monophasic pill	Consilient	30mcg	75mcg	Gestodene
Levest	21-day monophasic pill	Morningside	30mcg	150mcg	Levonogestrel
Microgynon 30	21-day monophasic pill	Bayer Schering	30mcg	150mcg	Levonogestrel
Ovranette	21-day monophasic pill	Wyeth	30mcg	150mcg	Levonogestrel
Rigevidon	21-day monophasic pill	Consilient	30mcg	150mcg	Levonogestrel
Loestrin 30	21-day monophasic pill	Galen	30mcg	1.5mg	Norethisterone acetate
Cilest	21-day monophasic pill	Janssen-Cilag	35mcg	250mcg	Norgestimate
Brevinor	21-day monophasic pill	Pharmacia	35mcg	500mcg	Norethisterone
Ovysmen	21-day monophasic pill	Janssen-Cilag	35mcg	500mcg	Norethisterone
Norimin	21-day monophasic pill	Pharmacia	35mcg	1mg	Norethisterone
Norinyl-1	21-day monophasic pill	Pharmacia	Mestranol 50mcg	1mg	Norethisterone

Table 7.2 Combined Everyday (ED) contraceptive pills

Combined pill name	Preparation	Manufacturer	Micrograms of oestrogen per pill	Micrograms of progestogen per pill	Type of progestogen
Microgynon ED	21-day monophasic pill with 7 inactive pills	Bayer Schering	30mcg	150mcg	Levonogestrel
Zoely	24-day monophasic pill	Bayer Schering	1.5mg Estradiol	2.5mg	Nomegestrol acetate
Femodene ED	21-day monophasic pill with 7 inactive pills	Bayer Schering	30mcg	75mcg	Gestodene

Triphasic pills

These follow a 21-day course and contain varying amounts of oestrogen (usually two different levels) throughout the packet but contain three different levels of progestogen, which are colour coded (e.g. Logynon, Synphase, Trinovum, Trinordiol, Tri-minulet, Triadene, TriRegol).

Everyday pills

Everyday (ED) pills are either monophasic or triphasic but follow a 28-day course. Twenty-one of these pills contain oestrogen and progestogen and seven are inactive containing no hormones (e.g. Femodene ED, Logynon ED, Microgynon ED, Qlaira).

Tailored regimens

Taking the combined pill continuously by tricycling or extending the combined pill for longer than 21 days or reducing the pill-free interval are unlicensed but can be beneficial. The only licensed combined pill with a reduced pill-free interval is Qlaira of two days and Zoely of four days.

Tricycling is where three cycles of monophasic pills are taken in a row without a break. The pill-free week is then taken at the end of the three months, and this is followed by a further three packets of pills. This reduces the number of pill-free weeks a woman has, so if she is complaining of problems in the pill-free week (e.g. headaches), then this can reduce the number of headaches she experiences in a year.

Side effects

- Nausea.
- Breast tenderness and swelling.
- Breakthrough bleeding.
- Depression.
- Changes in libido.
- Contact lenses may become uncomfortable – this is usually associated with hard lenses and high-dose pills.

Decision of choice of pill

When commencing the client on the combined pill, the risks along with the benefits should be discussed fully, so that the client is able to fully understand and weigh up the risks and benefits to them.

There are now six low-dose combined pills, all containing 20 micrograms of oestrogen. Loestrin 20 is a second-generation combined pill, and Mercilon, Gederal 20/150, Femodette, Millinette 20/75 and Sunya 20/75 are third-generation pills.

Yasmin is a new combined pill containing 3mg of drospirenone and 30 micrograms of ethinylestradiol. Yasmin has been found to significantly improve premenstrual symptoms such as water retention, acne and hirsutism (Daly and

Table 7.3 Phasic combined contraceptive pills

Combined pill name	Preparation	Manufacturer	Micrograms of oestrogen per pill	Micrograms of progestogen per pill	Type of progestogen
Triadene	6 pills 5 pills 10 pills	Bayer Schering	30mcg 40mcg 30mcg	50mcg 70mcg 100mcg	Gestodene
Logynon TreRegol	6 pills 5 pills 10 pills	Bayer Schering Consilient	30mcg 40mcg 30mcg	50mcg 75mcg 125mcg	Levonogestrel
Binovum	7 pills 14 pills	Janssen-Cilag	35mcg	500mcg 1mg	Norethisterone
Synphase	7 pills 9 pills 5 pills	Pharmacia	35mcg	500mcg 1mg 500mcg	Norethisterone
Trinovum	7 pills 7 pills 7 pills	Janssen-Cilag	35mcg	500mcg 750mcg 1mg	Northisterone

Table 7.4 Combined phasic Everyday (ED) contraceptive pills

Combined pill name	Preparation	Number of pills per cycle	Manufacturer	Micrograms of oestrogen per pill	Micrograms of progestogen per pill	Type of progestogen
Logynon ED	21-day pill with 7 inactive pills	6 pills	Bayer Schering	30mcg	50mcg	Levonogestrel
		5 pills		40mcg	75mcg	
		10 pills		30mcg	125mcg	
		7 inactive				
Qlaira	26-day pill with 2 inactive pills	2 pills	Bayer Schering	Estradiol Valerate 3mg		Dienogest
		5 pills		Estradiol Valerate 2mg	2mg	
		17 pills		Estradiol Valerate 2mg	3mg	
		2 pills		Estradiol Valerate 1mg		
		2 inactive				

Mansour, 2002). However, there is limited research on its effects on prothrombotic coagulation changes and, as a result, the incidence of venous thromboembolism, but it is now believed that the risk of venous thrombosis is similar to that of third-generation combined pills containing gestodene and desogestrel (FSRH, 2011a; PhVWP, 2011).

Qlaira is a new pill which contains estraodil valerate and dienogest, and has 26 active pills and two inactive. It has been found to reduce heavy menstrual bleeding and is the only combined pill licensed for this use. Qlaira's oestrogen is considered natural, and the progestogen dienogest is antiandrogenic. Qlaira has slightly different missed pill rules: a pill is missed if it is more than 12 hours late. If this happens, extra precautions will be required for nine days.

Zoely is a new combined pill which contains estradiol and a progestogen nomegestrol acetate. It is a 28-pill cycle, of which 24 are active pills and four inactive. A pill is considered missed if it is more than 12 hours late. After this point extra precautions will be required for seven days and, if these run into the inactive pills, these should be omitted and new active pills commenced.

Many women are prescribed Dianette for acne treatment which contains 2mg of cyproterone acetate and ethinylestradiol 35 micrograms and provides contraception. However, Dianette is not authorized for the sole purpose of contraception and should be discontinued after three to four menstrual cycles. There is evidence that Dianette has a higher incidence of venous thromboembolism than among women using low-dose oestrogen-containing combined pills (CSM, 2002). In 2013, France suspended the sale of Dianette over concerns that there were links with the deaths of four French women taking Diane 35 from venous thrombosis. The European Medicine Agency is currently reviewing the data and we await the outcome (EMA, 2013).

Many women are prescribed Dianette for the treatment of acne, but would not normally be put on the combined pill because their BMI is over 30 or they have another contra-indication. The reasons why a woman is taking Dianette should be reviewed and the risks discussed. Many new low-dose combined pills give excellent contraception and improve acne with a lower risk of venous thromboembolism.

The following risks should be discussed with all women considering the combined pill so that they are aware of the risks, and anyone who is contra-indicated is highlighted:

- Venous thromboembolism.
- Arterial disease.
- Breast cancer.
- Migraines.

Venous thromboembolism

There is a wide range of combined pills which may seem confusing when choosing a pill for a woman. The pill scare in October 1995 served to increase this chaos. Although the combined pill may only be prescribed by a doctor or independent prescriber or by certain nurses who are able to first issue under protocols, it is important for all nurses to understand the complexity of this issue so that they can advise women fully. The decision about which pill to prescribe will depend on the woman's medical and family history.

Table 7.5 Second-generation pills: pills containing Levonogestrel, Norethisterone or Ethynodiol

Oestrogen content	20mcg	30mcg	35mcg	Phasic
	Loestrin 20	Loestrin 30	Ovysmen	Trinovum
		Microgynon	Norimin	Logynon Logynon ED
		Ovranette	Brevinor	Binovum
		Rigevidon	Norinyl 1	
		Levest		

When explaining these risks it is important to remember that women who are not on the combined pill have a risk of venous thromboembolism of 5 to 10 in 100,000 per year and, even more importantly, the risk of venous thromboembolism in pregnancy is 60 in 100,000 per year. The risks of venous thromboembolism increase with age and obesity, and with other risk factors detailed below. Thus, while it is important to choose the right women to be on combined methods, it is also vital that the risks are explained clearly so that clients can understand these risks and the signs of venous thromboembolism.

The range of combined pills used today is mainly divided into two groups known as second- and third-generation pills. Pills in Table 7.5 are second-generation pills and contain the progestogen Levonorgestrel, Norethisterone or Ethynodiol, while the pills in Table 7.6 contain the progestogen Desogestrel or Gestodene and are known as third-generation pills. Yasmin is considered to have a similar risk of venous thromboembolism as third-generation combined pills.

The pill scare was related to three epidemiological studies (Jick *et al.*, 1995; WHO, 1995; Spitzer *et al.*, 1996) which showed that pills containing the progestogen Levonorgestrel, Norethisterone or Ethynodiol (which is converted to Norethisterone) have an incidence of venous thromboembolism for women of 15 per 100,000 per year. For women taking pills containing the progestogen Gestodene or Desogestrel the incidence doubles to 25 per 100,000 per year.

Table 7.6 Third-generation pills: pills containing Desogestrel or Gestodene

	Gestodene	Desogestrel	Drospirenone
30	Marvelon Gederal 30/150	Femodene Femodene ED Katya 30/75 Millinette 30/75	Yasmin
20	Mercilon Gederal 20/150	Femodette	

Research comparing Levonorgestrel and Desogestrel 30 microgram combined pills found that combined pills containing Levonorgestrel had the effect of opposing the oestrogenicity of the ethinyloestradiol and as a result lowered sex hormone-binding globulin. While combined pills containing the Desogestrel raised sex hormone-binding globulin, allowing these pills to have increased oestrogenic effects, this is associated with improvement of acne and increased prothrombotic coagulation changes (Guillebaud, 1999; Mackie et al., 2001).

More recent research has shown that the risk of venous thromboembolism is actually higher than originally thought. The risk of venous thromboembolism in second-generation combined pills is now thought to be 20 per 100,000 per year, and for third-generation combined pills it is 40 per 100,000 per year (PhVWP, 2011); this research only relates to combined pills. Research published on the combined contraceptive patch and ring is limited; however, a retrospective study has shown the risk of venous thromboembolism (VTE) with these methods to be twice the risk of second-generation combined pills (Lidegaard et al., 2012). The Clinical Effectiveness Unit has advised that there are limitations to this study, such as bias, family history of VTE and smoking, which makes it difficult to draw firm conclusions (FSRH, 2012c).

All of this research highlights the importance of selecting the right women for combined methods. No woman with a medical history of venous thromboembolism should be prescribed the combined pill; this is an absolute contra-indication. When assessing a woman's suitability for the pill, you should screen women for the following risk factors for venous thromboembolism:

- Family history of venous thromboembolism under the age of 45.
- Prominent varicose veins.
- Obesity (this is considered if the BMI is over 30 kgm^{-2}).
- Immobility (e.g. wheelchair bound).

When counselling a woman you should discuss the research and risk factors related to the combined pill. Any woman with any risk factor for venous thromboembolism should, after discussion with her, either be changed to another method of contraception or changed to a pill with a lower risk of venous thromboembolism. This could be a pill containing the progestogen Levonorgestrel, Norethisterone or Ethynodiol (see Table 7.5), as a low-dose pill should always be chosen. For the third-generation combined pill containing the progestogen Norgestimate (e.g. Cilest), there is currently insufficient information as to whether or not there is also an increased risk of venous thromboembolism.

Women with a family history of venous thromboembolism should be considered for screening for genetic susceptibility, since they may be carriers of the factor V Leiden mutation and thrombophilias; this will help ascertain if the woman is at risk of a venous thromboembolism. The incidence of the factor V Leiden mutation may range from 20 to 40 per cent in patients with recurrent venous thrombosis (Machin et al., 1995), which is why relevant screening is strongly advised. It is important to find out your employer's policy for screening, and where clients may be referred for this.

The Committee on Safety of Medicines advises that women who are intolerant to the second-generation pills but who are free of venous thromboembolism risk factors may, if willing to accept the small increased risk of venous thromboembolism, take the third-generation pill. Intolerance may be interpreted as minor side effects such as facial spots, acne or breakthrough bleeding which may be exacerbated by changing to a second-generation pill.

The risk of venous thromboembolism is highest in the first few months of commencement and this reduces to the same risk as non-users within weeks of discontinuation (FSRH, 2011a). This highlights the risks women put themselves under by stopping and starting the combined pill for a few months, which some women do under the misconception that they are reducing the risks of the condition. As health professionals it is important that we talk to our clients and answer questions about these risks, and teach clients when to return early.

Arterial disease

While it is important to assess women for risk factors for venous thromboembolism, it is equally important to assess for risk factors for arterial disease. Risk factors for arterial disease are as follows:

- Smoking.
- Diabetes mellitus.
- Mild to moderate hypertension; the combined pill is contra-indicated if the diastolic blood pressure is above 95mmHg.
- Family history of arterial disease under the age of 45.
- Obesity (BMI over 30kg m^{-2}).

You should discuss the risk factors for arterial disease with your client. If your client has more than one risk factor, then the combined pill will be contra-indicated, and if she is over 35 and has any risk factors the COC should be discontinued. If there is any family history of arterial disease, you should encourage your client to check her fasting lipids. Any family history of arterial disease under the age of 45 with no other risk factors necessitates relevant lipid screening. Combined pills containing the progestogens Gestodene, Desogestrel and Norgestimate appear to increase high-density lipoprotein (HDL) which may have a slightly more beneficial effect on lipid metabolism (Robinson, 1994) and hopefully coronary heart disease (Gillmer et al., 1996). One study (Lewis et al., 1996) on third-generation pills and risk of myocardial infarction concluded that, although they carried an increased risk of venous thromboembolism, this may be balanced with a reduced risk of myocardial infarction, but these results should be treated cautiously, especially with regard to smokers. However, at present further epidemiological data need to be accumulated before the potential protection against coronary heart disease can be fully assessed.

When choosing a suitable combined pill you should inform the woman of the risks so that she is able to make an informed decision. Medical histories should be updated regularly, and all issues discussed should be clearly documented, and backed up with relevant information.

Breast cancer

In June 1996 the Collaborative Group on Hormonal Factors in Breast Cancer published a study of re-analysis of world epidemiological data which related to 54 studies of over 53,000 women with breast cancer.

The re-analysis showed that there is a small increase in breast cancer risk for women taking the combined pill (Collaborative Group on Hormonal Factors in Breast Cancer, 1996a). The risk of breast cancer is when the woman is taking the combined pill, and during the 10 years following cessation there is a small increase in the relative risk of having breast cancer diagnosed. After 10 years following stopping the combined pill there is no increase in breast cancer risk. It was also found that women diagnosed with breast cancer who had used the COC had clinically less advanced cancers which were less likely to have spread beyond the breast compared with those in women who had not used the combined pill. The risks of breast cancer were not associated with the dose, duration or any type of hormone in the combined pill. The results were the same for all ethnic groups, and for those with family histories of breast cancer and different reproductive histories (Faculty of Family Planning and Reproductive Health Care of the Royal College of Obstetricians and Gynaecologists, 1996). Because breast cancer incidence increases with age, so the cumulative excess risk increases with increasing age for women starting and 10 years after stopping the combined pill.

However, in 2002 studies by the United States Centers for Disease Control showed no increased combined pill-related risk of breast cancer (Marchbanks *et al.*, 2002). Studies in 2010 also showed no increased increased risk of breast cancer (Vessey *et al.*, 2010).

The Faculty of Sexual and Reproductive Healthcare's advice is that any risk of breast cancer associated with the combined pill is small and will reduce after stopping (FSRH, 2011a). In spite of this, the consultation provides a good opportunity to encourage women to self-examine their breasts and to explain what to look for when doing so.

Migraines

It is important to ask all women about their headache and migraine history. Many women experience headaches which are actually undiagnosed migraines, so it is important to identify which women are at an increased risk of an ischaemic stroke if they are given the combined pill. You will need to ask explicit questions as the client may not be aware of the significance of her headaches; you may also find that women who are already taking the combined pills and experiencing migraines with aura are unaware of the risks. Questions like 'Have you ever had a headache or migraine where you have experienced problems with your vision or had numbness or tingling?' usually help to reveal any past history. If a woman suffers from one of the following types of migraine and she is already taking the combined pill or wishing to commence it then she will have an absolute contra-indication UKMEC 4 to it and will need to be reviewed by a doctor:

1   Migraine with aura: this is where there are focal neurological symptoms preceding the headaches. A woman may experience loss of vision or visual disturbances, numbness or tingling; this is UKMEC 4.
2   Migraine without aura where a woman has more than one additional risk factor for an ischaemic stroke. These risk factors are being aged 35 and over, diabetes mellitus, family history of arterial disease below the age of 45, hyperlipidaemia, hypertension, migraine, obesity (defined as a body mass index over 30), smoking and the combined pill. This is UKMEC 3/4.
3   Migraines which are severe and last longer than 72 hours.

4   Migraine which is treated with ergot derivatives.
5   Past history of migraine more than five years previously with aura.

Women with migraines who are taking the combined pill have a two- to four-fold increased risk of an ischaemic stroke compared to those not using the combined pill (FSRH, 2009a), so it is important to explain why you are not prescribing the method they have requested so that they are not given it in the future.

Women who suffer from these types of migraines can use the progestogen-only pill, injectable contraception, IUS or any other non-hormonal method of contraception.

How to take the combined pill

The combined 21-day pill should be commenced on the first day of your client's period. When she starts the pill on the first day of her period no additional precautions are required; these instructions are the same for all 21-day pills whether they are monophasic, biphasic or triphasic. If the pill is commenced at any other time in the cycle additional precautions are required for seven days. You should encourage your client to take her pills at the same time each day. Once 21 days of pills have been taken then she should have a seven-day break where no pills are taken; this is known as the pill-free week. Following the seven-day break she should restart the pill on day 8. Each packet of pills will always be commenced on the same day of the week the first packet is commenced.

Loss of efficacy of the combined pill

The combined pill's effectiveness is reduced by the following:

■   Missed pills – if your client forgets to take her pill and is more than 24 hours late.
■   Vomiting – if your client vomits within three hours of taking the pill.
■   Severe diarrhoea.
■   Drugs which are enzyme inducers (see Table 7.7).

Loss of efficacy through drug interaction

Liver enzyme-inducing drugs

If your client is given an enzyme-inducing drug like Rifampicin on a long-term basis then alternative contraception is recommended (e.g. the injectable Depoprovera given at 10-week intervals or an intrauterine device). Women wishing to continue with the combined pill while taking anticonvulsant or barbiturate drugs which affect the efficacy of the COC will need to change to a pill containing a higher concentration of oestrogen – at least 50mg – and tricycle (this means taking three monophasic packets of pills in a row without a break). The pill-free week may also be reduced to four days to increase the efficacy of the pill. If breakthrough bleeding occurs then the oestrogen content of the pill should be increased to 60 to 90mg once abnormal pathology has been excluded. It takes four weeks for the liver's

Table 7.7 Enzyme-inducing drugs which reduce the efficacy of combined methods. Enzyme-inducing drugs reduce the efficacy of the combined methods by the induction of liver enzymes, which increase the metabolism of the combined methods.

Drug type	Drug
Anticonvulsants	Carbamazepine
	Esilcarbamazepine
	Oxcarbazepine
	Phenytoin
	Perampanel
	Phenobarbital
	Primidone
	Topiramate
	Rifinamide
Antitubercle	Rifamycins (e.g. Rifampicin, Rifabutin)
Antiretroviral: Protease inhibitors	Ritonavir
	Ritonavir boosted atazanavir
	Ritonavir boosted tipranavir
	Ritonavir boosted saquinavir
	Nelfinaavir, Darunavir, Fosamprenavir, Lopinavir
Antiretroviral: Non-nucleoside reverse transcriptase inhibitors	Nevirapine
	Efavirenz
Other enzyme-inducing drugs	Modafinil
	Bosentan
	Aprepitant
	Sugammadex
Homeopathic	St Johns Wort

excretory function to return to normal once liver enzyme drugs have been discontinued. It is advisable to allow eight weeks following cessation before a lower combined pill is commenced.

Missed pill rules

Many women either forget or are given little information about missed pill rules so it is a good idea to check frequently that your client is up to date with current guidelines and has relevant written information to back this up. The importance of this information is often underestimated by both women and professionals; however, as poor compliance will affect the efficacy of the combined pill, it is essential that missed pill rules are covered (Fig. 7.1).

If your client forgets a pill but it is 24 hours (but no longer than 48 hours) from when she normally takes it, then she should take it immediately and no additional precautions are required.

If your client forgets two or more pills and it is now more than 48 hours late then the missed pill should be taken and the remaining pills taken at the normal time and

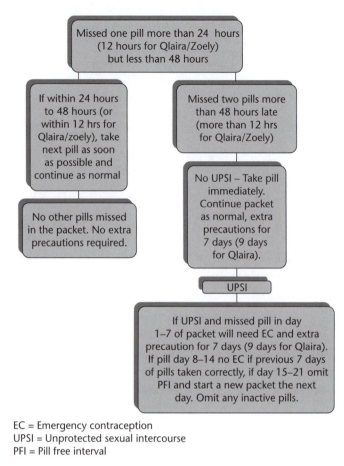

Missed one pill more than 24 hours (12 hours for Qlaira/Zoely) but less than 48 hours

If within 24 hours to 48 hours (or within 12 hrs for Qlaira/zoely), take next pill as soon as possible and continue as normal

No other pills missed in the packet. No extra precautions required.

Missed two pills more than 48 hours late (more than 12 hrs for Qlaira/Zoely)

No UPSI – Take pill immediately. Continue packet as normal, extra precautions for 7 days (9 days for Qlaira).

UPSI

If UPSI and missed pill in day 1–7 of packet will need EC and extra precaution for 7 days (9 days for Qlaira). If pill day 8–14 no EC if previous 7 days of pills taken correctly, if day 15–21 omit PFI and start a new packet the next day. Omit any inactive pills.

EC = Emergency contraception
UPSI = Unprotected sexual intercourse
PFI = Pill free interval

Figure 7.1 Missed combined oral contraceptive pill guidelines

extra precautions will now be required for seven days . If the pill-free week runs into this time then this should be omitted and the next packet commenced straight away if it is a monphasic pill (see Table 7.1). If the pill is biphasic or triphasic and the pill-free week runs into this time then the pill-free week should be omitted, but the client will need to take enough pills from the end of another packet which match the end of the present packet in colour and dose, and take additional precautions for seven days following the missed pill. If the pill is an Everyday (ED) pill and the seven days of additional precautions required run into the end of the packet, the seven inactive pills should be omitted and the next packet commenced straight away.

If the pills are missed in the first seven days of the packet and there has been unprotected sexual intercourse in the pill-free interval or in the first week of the packet, then emergency contraception should be considered. If the pills are missed in the second week of the packet days 8 to 14 then emergency contraception is not required if the pills have not been missed for the previous seven days of the packet. Extra precautions will be required for the next seven days of pills, however.

If your client vomits within three hours of taking the pill or suffers from very severe diarrhoea then the combined pill will not be effective and additional precautions will be required during this time and for a further seven days once these symptoms have been resolved. Again, if this runs into the pill-free week then this should be omitted and, if it is a monophasic pill, the next packet resumed immediately. If the pill is a biphasic or triphasic pill then your client will need to take enough pills from the end of another packet which match in dose and colour.

Women are safe to have sexual intercourse in the seven-day pill-free week, as long as they do not extend this gap. If your client does extend this gap she is at risk of ovulating and pregnancy. If she forgets the last pill of her packet she should be advised to count that as the first day of the pill-free week and only have a further six pill-free days. If she forgets to restart her next packet on time and has had an eight-day pill-free interval then her pills will not be contraceptively effective until she has taken seven days of pills; in the meantime she will need to use additional contraceptive precautions. If she is more than one pill late in restarting her packet then emergency contraception may be required.

Initial consultation

Time spent covering the risks and missed pill rules of the combined pill may alleviate future problems and save you and your client time and anxiety in the future. Many women attend having made their contraceptive choice; this does not mean that they do not have absolute contra-indications to the combined pill, so a careful medical history of the client and her family is vital. Often a change in contraception is precipitated by unprotected sexual intercourse or an accident with another contraceptive method, so it is important to establish whether emergency contraception is required. Details about the last menstrual period should be obtained, as this will help to build a picture of whether there is any possibility of pregnancy. If there has been unprotected sexual intercourse then the client may already be pregnant, and a pregnancy test may need to be performed. Unprotected sexual intercourse is often abbreviated to UPSI.

CASE STUDY 7.1

A 23-year-old woman consults requesting the combined pill. She appears aloof and distant, answering questions with limited replies and poor eye contact. When asked about previous contraception, she says she has recently had two years with no contraception, but has been having sexual intercourse. Eventually with time she says 'that things have changed in her relationship' and although she wanted to get pregnant this is no longer the case. There is now an opportunity to discuss the problems within her relationship and she decides to see if her partner will attend for couple counselling.

Look carefully at how your client is sitting, her body language and listen to how she is talking to you and what she is saying. Both men and women can tell you a great deal about themselves from their body language and the feelings they portray.

The risks of the combined pill should be discussed. It is important that your client is aware of the signs of these risks and when to attend early. If your client experiences any of the following problems she should seek medical attention:

- Pain and swelling in the calf of her leg.
- Chest pain.
- Shortness of breath.
- Increasing headaches.
- Headaches with speech or visual disturbances.
- Pain, tingling or weakness in her arm or leg.
- Jaundice.
- Severe abdominal pain.
- Post-coital bleeding or any prolonged bleeding.

Basic observations should be performed like blood pressure, weight and height. You should calculate your client's BMI, which will help to exclude any absolute contra-indications. Details of previous contraception should be covered with any problems your client encountered, as this will help you choose a suitable pill for your client.

Missed pill rules and emergency contraception should be covered, along with when to commence the pill and when efficacy is reduced. Often women do not know how long after unprotected sexual intercourse emergency contraception may be given, and even if they never need to use this information they may have a friend who does. What is often forgotten is that women learn a great deal from their friends but sometimes this information is inaccurate; on many occasions a client's visit is prompted by a friend.

During your history taking you should eliminate any absolute contra-indications to the pill. If there are signs of vaginal infection then appropriate screening should be performed; if this is unavailable she should be referred to a genito-urinary medicine clinic. If your client is experiencing any post-coital bleeding (often abbreviated to PCB), she should be referred for a cervical smear along with a bimanual examination. PCB can be a sign of infection, cervical ectopy, polyps or malignancy. If there are no problems then you should record previous cervical cytology and discuss with your client when this needs to be repeated. Women who have not had a cervical smear often fear being forced to have a smear, but if there are no clinical problems then this may be deferred to a convenient time. If your client has any sexual anxieties or problems then she may feel comfortable to discuss them nearer the end of the consultation. Giving her time and allowing her to talk will help enable her to approach this difficult subject.

The consultation is a prime time to discuss disease prevention. If your client has a family history of heart disease then it can be useful to discuss blood lipid screening, diet and smoking. You should discuss with your client how the risks of the pill are increased by smoking; if she ceases smoking then these risks will reduce to the same as a non-smoker. It is also a good opportunity to promote breast awareness, and preconceptual screening such as sickle cell screening and rubella status. Although your client may have no intention at the moment of becoming pregnant this is often a good time to perform screening in case immunization for rubella is required.

Women often underestimate the need for protection against sexually transmitted infections and HIV. There is a belief among many men and women that 'it won't happen to me', and it is often difficult for a nurse to approach this subject when clients are unable to accept that this is an issue. However, you will need to discuss safer sex and the use of condoms with your client as the pill offers no protection against STIs and HIV and she may not have considered this subject.

Discuss with your client initial problems she may encounter and how to alleviate these (e.g. breakthrough bleeding and nausea; see section on 'Problems encountered') and when you will need to see her again. It is important to inform your client of any potential side effects as this will help alleviate anxiety. Most side effects normally settle within the first three months, so it is always worth continuing with a pill rather than changing to another pill where the symptoms may be perpetuated. A woman commencing the combined pill should be seen in three months' time. If there are no problems then she should be seen every six months from then onward.

Finally, everything you have discussed with your client should be backed up with up-to-date written information. Often men and women do not read leaflets so you cannot rely on just giving them the leaflets – you will need to say it verbally as well. It is also possible that your client is unable to read, but may not be prepared to admit this, or that English is not her first language. If this is the case try to obtain leaflets in her first language. You should also give telephone numbers where clients can obtain advice and emergency contraception.

The points to be covered at initial consultation are summarized in Box 7.1.

CASE STUDY 7.2

A 26-year-old woman consults having been on the combined pill for five years. She complains of increased headaches and in discussion she says that she is experiencing visual problems with the headaches. When she reads when suffering a headache she finds that she is unable to see words in the text and has been getting some tingling in her tongue. It is explained to the client that what she is experiencing are focal migraines and these are an absolute contra-indication with the combined pill and put her at an increased risk of a stroke. After discussion with the client other methods of contraception are suggested; she decides to try the progestogen pill and is given Cerazette while she considers other methods. She is now unable to take the combined pill, patch or ring, as her headaches are focal migraines and this is an absolute contra-indication to these methods, since they contain oestrogen, but she may be given progestogen methods.

Subsequent visits

At subsequent visits it is important to ascertain whether your client has had any problems of any kind, which may include increasing headaches or migraines. This may be performed by asking open-ended questions like 'How have you got on with your pill?' Allow her time to answer questions. Often clients report that they have no problems, but just as they are about to leave they mention that they have had visual problems with a headache or forgotten a pill and not used extra precautions.

Routine observations of weight and blood pressure should be performed. Information about the last menstrual period will help eliminate any risk of pregnancy and also checks that she is taking her pills correctly. Questions to ask include: Is your client's cervical smear up to date? Is she experiencing any problems with her periods or sexual intercourse? Is your client aware of missed pill rules and emergency contraception? Does she have up-to-date information on her pills? Does she have any anxieties or questions?

BOX 7.1

Points to be covered at initial consultation

- Full medical history.
- Family medical history.
- Basic observations: BP, weight, height, BMI.
- Has the client had unprotected sexual intercourse and is she in need of emergency contraception or already pregnant?
- Cervical cytology and breast awareness.
- Risks of the combined pill, and when to seek medical attention.
- Missed pill rules.
- Emergency contraception.
- Safer sex.
- Leaflets on the COC and emergency contraception given to client.
- Relevant telephone numbers for advice.

If your client has no problems then a prescription for six months' supply may be given. It is a good idea to encourage your client to return in five months' time so that she has a spare (emergency) packet of pills. You could also ask if she needs a supply of condoms, and whether she is aware of how to apply a condom or does she need to be taught. If your client is a non-smoker and has no contra-indications or complications then she may continue to take the pill until she is peri-menopausal.

The points to be covered at subsequent visits are summarized in Box 7.2.

BOX 7.2

Points to be covered at subsequent visits

- Update of medical and family history.
- Basic observation: BP, weight, height.
- Date of last menstrual period, has she had any problems with her pill?
- Is her cervical smear due?
- Is she breast aware?
- Do missed pill rules need revision?
- Safer sex: is she at risk?
- Has she got up-to-date leaflets on the COC and emergency contraception?
- Have relevant telephone numbers for advice been given?

ACTIVITY

Do you know where your clients can obtain contraception and emergency contraception in your area when you are not working?

Reasons for breakthrough bleeding (BTB) with the COC

It is not unusual for women to have breakthrough bleeding (BTB) in the first two months of starting a combined pill; this can be alarming for women if they are not warned of this possibility beforehand. It is important that women continue to take their pill, as the bleeding usually stops after two to three packets and, providing all the pills have been taken correctly, contraceptive efficacy will not be affected. If bleeding continues beyond three packets of pills then the cause should be investigated. It may be due to:

- Missed pills.
- Diarrhoea or vomiting.
- Drugs which interact with the COC and affect the efficacy (e.g. enzyme-inducing drugs).
- Disease of the cervix (e.g. cervical cancer, sexually transmitted infections such as chlamydia).
- Pregnancy.
- Diet (e.g. vegetarians).
- The dose level of the pill may not suit the client.

When excluding all possible causes of BTB it is vital to take a detailed history from the woman. This will help ascertain what the cause is and whether contraceptive efficacy has been reduced and emergency contraception is indicated. The type of pill preparation should not be changed until all causes have been excluded. If the BTB is caused by the dose of pill preparation then a pill with a different or higher dose of progestogen should be prescribed.

PROBLEMS ENCOUNTERED WHILE ON THE PILL

Breakthrough bleeding

Breakthrough bleeding may be due to disease of the cervix such as cervical neoplasia or a sexually transmitted infection such as chlamydia, so appropriate screening may need to be performed. Pregnancy may cause breakthrough bleeding so this may need to be excluded. If your client has missed pills or had diarrhoea or vomiting then there may be loss of effectiveness of the pill and bleeding. Drugs which cause loss of efficacy of the pill may cause BTB (see Table 7.7). The client may need to find alternative contraception or change to a higher oestrogen content pill. Women who are vegetarians occasionally have BTB, as their enterohepatic circulation may be affected by their bowel flora. Occasionally women who have had extensive bowel surgery may suffer BTB because the absorption of the pill is impaired.

Breakthrough bleeding may occur because your client has not been on the pill for sufficient duration. It is not unusual to experience BTB in the first few months of taking the pill; this usually disappears, so it is important to continue with the pill. However, if bleeding is experienced and she has taken the pill for three to four packets with no improvement, and all other causes of BTB have been excluded, then the dosage or type of pill may need to changed. The pill may be changed as the dose may be too low; this can be done by choosing a pill with a higher oestrogen content or one with a different progestogen component. It may be necessary to prescribe a pill containing 50mg of oestrogen.

Your client forgets to take her pill

It is useful to discuss with your client why she thinks she forgets her pills; this may be because of problems in a relationship, or she may subconsciously desire a pregnancy. If she forgets her pill it can be a useful reminder to keep the pill next to her alarm clock, or near the coffee or tea jar or next to her toothbrush, or she could set her phone to remind her. It is a good idea to suggest that she carries a spare packet of the pill in her purse so that if she has forgotten to take her pill she is likely to have a packet with her. Alarm watches and personal computers and mobile phones can be set to act as a reminder. There are apps that can be downloaded to help remind clients about pill taking.

Complaints of nausea

If your client complains of nausea she should make sure that the pill is taken after eating. If this continues she may need to change to a different type of pill or one containing less oestrogen.

Breast tenderness

If this is experienced in the first three months then usually the symptoms resolve. However, if your client complains of breast tenderness her breasts should be examined. Evening primrose oil and vitamin B6 can help relieve symptoms if taken continuously. If symptoms persist it may be necessary to change to a pill containing lower levels of oestrogen and progestogen or a different type of progestogen.

Increased spots and acne

Try changing to a pill with a different progestogen.

Weight gain

Often clients complain of increased weight. Initially they may have a small weight gain, but usually weight gain is due to changes in diet and exercise.

Vaginal dryness and loss of libido

Try to discuss with your client any anxieties or problems she may have in the relationship which may be causing this problem. Try changing to a different pill.

Headaches prior to periods

It is important to check that these headaches do not cause focal disturbances, as this would be an absolute contra-indication to the pill. It may be useful for your client to keep a diary of her headaches and when they occur. If they occur in the pill-free week then tricycling will reduce the number of headaches. Headaches in the pill-free week are usually because the hormone levels have dropped.

THE COMBINED CONTRACEPTIVE PATCH

Introduction and history

The first combined contraceptive patch was launched onto the UK market in 2003. The only combined contraceptive patch currently available is known as Evra from Janssen-Cilag.

Explanation of the method

Evra releases 150 micrograms of norelgestromin and 20 micrograms of ethinylestradiol per 24 hours; norelgestromin is the primary active metabolite of norgestimate (the progestogen contained in the combined pill Cilest). Evra is a transdermal patch which lasts for seven days. The patches are used for three weeks consecutively, with a new patch applied each week. This period is followed by a patch-free week of seven days in the fourth week where a withdrawal bleed occurs. Evra prevents pregnancy by inhibiting ovulation, altering cervical mucus so that it is impenetrable to sperm and by making the endometrium unfavourable to implantation.

Efficacy

The efficacy for Evra is over 99 per cent with careful and consistent use. However, with less careful use it can be 91 per cent (FSRH, 2011a). In women whose weight is equal to or greater than 90kg, contraceptive efficacy may be decreased (Janssen-Cilag, 2003; Zieman et al., 2002).

UKMEC 4 unacceptable health risk: absolute contra-indication

Contra-indications are the same for Evra as for the combined pill:

- Pregnancy.
- Breast-feeding.
- Less than six weeks post-partum.
- Undiagnosed vaginal or uterine bleeding.
- Past or present venous thrombosis.
- Past or present arterial thrombosis.
- Cardiovascular and ischaemic heart disease.
- Complicated pulmonary hypertension, atrial fibrilation and subacute bacterial endocarditis.
- Migraine with aura.
- Cerebrovascular accident and transient ischaemic attacks.
- Active disease of the liver (e.g. malignancy, history of cholestatic jaundice, impaired liver function tests, acute viral hepatitis, severe cirrhosis).
- Current breast cancer.
- Systemic lupus erythematosus with positive antiphospholipid antibodies.
- Raynaud's disease with lupus anticoagulant; if present this will increase coagulation.
- Stevens–Johnson syndrome.
- Acute pancreatitis.
- Four weeks before major surgery or leg surgery.
- Known thrombogenic mutations such as Factor V Leiden, Prothrombin mutation, Protein S and Protein C, and Antithrombin deficiencies.
- Severe diabetes mellitus with complications such as retinopathy, neuropathy, vascular disease.
- Smokers over the age of 35.
- Hypertension with a diastolic over 95mm Hg.

UKMEC 3 risks outweigh the benefits of using method: relative contra-indication

- Obesity (body mass index (BMI) over 35kg m^{-2}).
- Lipid disorders and diseases where high-density lipoprotein (HDL) is reduced (e.g. diabetes, hypertension).

- Migraine without aura.
- Past history of migraine with aura at any age.
- Carriers of known gene mutations linked to breast cancer BRCAS 1.
- Past history of breast cancer in the last five years.
- History of cholestasis with a combined method.
- Gallstones.
- Diseases whose drug treatment affects the efficacy of the combined pill (e.g. tuberculosis, epilepsy).
- Family history of arterial or venous disease in a first-degree relative below the age of 45.

Side effects

- Nausea.
- Breast tenderness and swelling.
- Headaches.
- Application site skin reactions.

How to take the combined contraceptive patch

Evra should be commenced initially on the first day of a woman's menstrual period. The patch should be applied to clean, dry, hairless skin and held down firmly for about 10 seconds until firmly attached. The site of the patch should be changed each week. The first patch should remain *in situ* for seven days. A new patch should be applied on day 8 and this should remain *in situ* for a further seven days. A third patch should be applied on day 15 and this remains in place until day 22 when the patch is removed and the patch-free interval begins for seven days. During these seven days a withdrawal bleed occurs. A new patch is then applied on day 8. Research has shown breakthrough bleeding with Evra to be low (Sibai *et al.*, 2002).

Loss of efficacy of the combined contraceptive patch

The combined contraceptive patch's effectiveness is reduced by:

- The patch coming off or partly detaching, or delays in changing or commencing the patch.
- Drugs which are enzyme inducers (see Table 7.7).

Loss of efficacy through drug interaction

The effectiveness of Evra is reduced with enzyme-inducing drugs (see Table 7.7).

Missed patch rules

If a patch detaches for fewer than 48 hours then it should be reapplied or replaced with a new patch immediately and no additional contraception is necessary. The next patch should be applied on the usual change day. If the patch has been detached for 48 hours or more, then a new contraceptive patch should be applied and a new cycle commenced; in these cases, additional contraception is required for seven days.

If patch change days are delayed by fewer than 48 hours at the start of the patch cycle, efficacy may be reduced. If this happens, a new patch should be applied immediately and alternative contraception used for seven days. This will mean that the patch change day will be altered. If there is a prolonged delay (more than 48 hours) in the change of patch at the start of the patch cycle, emergency contraception may be required.

If the patch change day is delayed in the middle cycle for one to two days (up to 48 hours) the client should apply a new patch immediately. The next patch should be applied on the usual patch change day and, if the patch has been worn correctly for the seven preceding days, no additional contraception is required. If the patch is delayed by more than two days (48 hours or more) the client may not be protected. In this situation, the client should commence a new patch immediately, meaning that there is a new change day; alternative contraception will also be required for seven days.

Sexuality and anxieties

Contraceptive patches offer women an extremely useful alternative. Mobile phones can be set with reminders to help a woman to remember to change her patch. Many women are used to using patches in the form of nicotine patches to help stop smoking, so will find the contraceptive patch a welcome concept. Evra may be perceived by young women as trendy and fashionable.

THE COMBINED CONTRACEPTIVE RING

Introduction and history

The combined contraceptive ring was launched in the UK in January 2009 but has been available in the USA since 2002. It is manufactured by Organon under the name NuvaRing.

Explanation of the method

NuvaRing is a non-biodegradable latex-free combined contraceptive vaginal ring which releases 120 micrograms of the progestogen etonogestrel and 15 micrograms of the oestrogen ethinylestradiol every 24 hours and remains in the vagina for three weeks. After this it is removed for one week, during which time a withdrawal bleed will occur, and a new ring is inserted. NuvaRing is 4mm thick and 54mm in diameter, and can be inserted into the vagina and removed by women themselves.

NuvaRing prevents pregnancy by inhibiting ovulation, altering cervical mucus so that it is impenetrable to sperm and by making the endometrium unfavourable to implantation.

Efficacy

The efficacy for the NuvaRing is over 99 per cent with careful and consistent use; however, with less careful use it can be 91 per cent (FSRH, 2011a).

UKMEC 4 unacceptable health risk: absolute contra-indication

Contra-indications are the same for NuvaRing as for the combined pill:

■ Conditions which will increase the expulsion of the ring (e.g. prolapse of cervix, cystocele, rectocele, severe or chronic constipation).
■ Pregnancy.
■ Breast-feeding.
■ Less than six weeks post-partum.
■ Undiagnosed vaginal or uterine bleeding.
■ Past or present venous thrombosis.
■ Past or present arterial thrombosis.
■ Cardiovascular and ischaemic heart disease.
■ Complicated pulmonary hypertension, atrial fibrilation and subacute bacterial endocarditis.
■ Migraine with aura.
■ Cerebrovascular accident and transient ischaemic attacks.
■ Active disease of the liver (e.g. malignancy, history of cholestatic jaundice, impaired liver function tests, acute viral hepatitis, severe cirrhosis).
■ Current breast cancer.
■ Systemic lupus erythematosus with positive antiphospholipid antibodies.
■ Raynaud's disease with lupus anticoagulant; if present this will increase coagulation.
■ Stevens–Johnson syndrome.
■ Acute pancreatitis.
■ Four weeks before major surgery or leg surgery.
■ Known thrombogenic mutations such as Factor V Leiden, Prothrombin mutation, Protein S and Protein C and Antithrombin deficiencies.
■ Severe diabetes mellitus with complications such as retinopathy, neuropathy, vascular disease.
■ Smokers over the age of 35.
■ Hypertension with a diastolic over 95mm Hg.

UKMEC 3 risks outweigh the benefits of using method: relative contra-indication

■ Obesity (body mass index (BMI) over 35kg m^{-2}).
■ Lipid disorders and diseases where high-density lipoprotein (HDL) is reduced (e.g. diabetes, hypertension).
■ Migraine without aura.
■ Past history of migraine with aura at any age.
■ Carriers of known gene mutations linked to breast cancer BRCAS 1.
■ Past history of breast cancer in the last five years.

- History of cholestasis with a combined method.
- Gallstones.
- Diseases whose drug treatment affects the efficacy of the combined pill (e.g. tuberculosis, epilepsy).
- Family history of arterial or venous disease in a first-degree relative below the age of 45.

How to use the combined contraceptive ring

NuvaRing should be inserted into the vagina on the first day of the period and left *in situ* for three weeks. This should be followed by a seven-day ring-free week after which a new ring should be inserted for a further three weeks. NuvaRing will be effective in preventing pregnancy if started on the first day of the period. If it is started from day 2 of the cycle onwards, extra precautions will be required for seven days. During the ring-free week women should experience a withdrawal bleed. Women should be shown how to remove and fit the ring. The ring should be compressed and inserted into the vagina; it does not need to be in a particular position but should feel comfortable. To remove the ring, women should loop their finger around it and pull it out. The ring should be disposed of in household waste.

The ring's position should be checked prior to intercourse to ensure that it is correctly positioned. NuvaRing may be left *in situ* during sexual intercourse and if tampons are used.

Prior to dispensing NuvaRing it is kept in a pharmacy fridge at temperatures between 2 to 8 degrees Celsius and can be stored this way for 40 months. Once NuvaRing is dispensed it can be left out of the fridge for four months, but this means that only three months can be dispensed at a time. When the three-month pack is dispensed the date should be written on it and the life span outside the fridge discussed. Women should keep their NuvaRings at room temperature once dispensed.

Loss of efficacy of the combined contraceptive ring

As the etonogestrel and ethinyestradiol in the ring are absorbed via the vagina they avoid the first pass metabolism of oral combined methods so will not be affected by gastrointestinal disturbances and malabsorption disorders from the upper bowel. However, the antifungal drug miconazole has been shown to increase the release of etonogestrel and ethinyestradiol and result in higher serum levels. Antifungals do not appear to reduce contraceptive efficacy; however, they are associated with increases in ring breakages (FSRH, 2009c).

Loss of efficacy through drug interaction

The effectiveness of NuvaRing is reduced with enzyme-inducing drugs (see Table 7.7).

Missed ring rules

The contraceptive ring's efficacy can be reduced if the ring is left out of the vagina for more than 48 hours, and if this occurs extra precautions should be taken for seven days. If this is in the first week of the cycle, emergency contraception will be required for any unprotected sexual intercourse. If the ring has been left out of the vagina and it is in the second and third week of use and the ring has been used consistently for the past seven days, then extra precautions will be required for only seven days. If this happens in week 3, the woman can insert a new ring and miss her ring-free week and use extra precautions for seven days.

If the ring-free week is extended because the woman forgets to insert a new ring by less than 48 hours, no extra precautions are required. However, if the ring-free week is extended by more than 48 hours then a new ring should be inserted and emergency contraception will be required for any unprotected sexual intercourse; extra precautions should be advised for seven days.

The future

In the future the way we prescribe combined hormones is likely to develop further. Research is underway on a combined monthly injectable contraceptive. Greater choices in the way we give hormones will appeal to women and increase compliance. With methods like patches and rings, text message reminders can be set up on mobile phones to remind women to change their method, and this idea is often attractive to young women.

SELF-ASSESSMENT QUESTIONS

Answers and discussion at the end of the chapter.

1 In what situations would extra precautions be required with the combined pill?
2 Name four beneficial effects the combined pill has on a woman's body.
3 What are the main concerns or myths about the combined pill that women worry about and how would you answer their questions?
4 Name the second-generation pills missing in the following table (see Table 7.5 for answers).

Oestrogen content	20mcg	30mcg	35mcg	Phasic

5   Name the third-generation pills missing in the following table (see Table 7.6 for answers).

	Gestodene	Desogestrel	Drospirenone
30			3mg
20			

Sexuality and anxieties

The combined pill has given women greater freedom over their bodies and fertility, allowing them to choose when they wish to become pregnant. However, this has drawbacks – women often find the decision to stop the pill and try to conceive a dilemma. They hope to find the perfect time to become pregnant which will probably never happen, and at the same time they may feel that time is running out as their body clock ticks ominously away. For some women the pill is too effective; they would like to become pregnant and not have to make the decision.

Women who frequently forget to take their pill may have a subconscious desire to become pregnant, but it may be difficult for them to admit to this feeling. Some women have been brought up to believe that sexual intercourse is only for procreation and by taking the pill they are preventing pregnancy, resulting in loss of enjoyment of sexual intercourse.

Women may blame the combined pill for problems which are unrelated to it. Frequent changes of type of pill may indicate an underlying problem. Given time and an empathetic approach these may be vocalized.

Some women feel an enormous amount of guilt for enjoying sexual intercourse with the protection of the pill, and this guilt is often expressed by women who feel that the pill will make them infertile. They feel that there is some divine retribution for being on the pill, and this has been compounded by pill scares. Recently, women and their partners will have read and listened to alarmist articles and news reports in the UK about the pill; the anxiety this has engendered has been enormous. Articles entitled 'The pill can kill' have meant that many women now have a negative image of the combined pill which does not reflect its true properties. Women are often surprised by how small the risk of venous thromboembolism and breast cancer actually is. There is also a belief that there should be no risk attached to the pill. This unrealistic view fails to acknowledge the risks of pregnancy, and also the everyday risks we all automatically accept, such as driving a car or smoking. It is therefore important that we educate and inform women about the risks of the combined pill, and are able to confront the anxieties and alarm they may have in a calm and responsible manner (Editorial, 1996). It will be some time before men and women feel as confident about the pill as they did prior to the pill scare.

ANSWERS TO SELF-ASSESSMENT QUESTIONS

1 *In what situations would extra precautions be required with the combined pill?*

Extra precautions are required when the pill's effectiveness is decreased. This may be due to a pill being taken more than 48 hours after its normal time. Extra precautions are also required if the woman has severe diarrhoea or vomiting, or commences a drug which reduces the efficacy of the pill like an enzyme-inducing drug (e.g. Rifampicin).

2 *Name four beneficial effects the combined pill has on a woman's body.*

The combined pill reduces the risk of endometrial and ovarian cancer. It reduces benign breast disease, dysmenorrhoea and menorrhagia, and as a result of this reduces the incidence of iron deficiency anaemia. There is less risk of ectopic pregnancy and a reduction of functional ovarian cysts. Psychologically the combined pill gives women assurance against unwanted pregnancy and relief from possible disabling premenstrual symptoms.

3 *What are the main concerns or myths about the combined pill that women worry about and how would you answer their questions?*

One of the major concerns women wish to discuss about the combined pill is that 'the pill makes you infertile'. This is a myth. The pill is completely reversible and does not cause infertility; however, no one knows whether they can become pregnant until they do so. A study on primary infertility and the combined pill (Bagwell *et al.*, 1995) concluded that the COC was associated with a lower incidence of primary infertility.

Another concern women have is related to the length of time they take the pill; they feel 'you should give your body a rest from the pill'. There is no medical reason to stop the pill. Often when women do stop to have a rest this is when they accidentally become pregnant, causing them great anguish.

Many women are concerned that the pill is dangerous. In fact the combined pill is a very safe and effective form of contraception. It is not dangerous unless there is a medical contra-indication. Smoking is more of a health risk than taking the pill, which is why smokers cannot take the pill after the age of 35.

8 THE PROGESTOGEN-ONLY PILL

- Introduction and history
- The progestogen-only pill
- Sexuality and anxieties

INTRODUCTION AND HISTORY

The progestogen-only pill used to be referred to as the 'mini-pill', which tends to give women the impression that it is of a low contraceptive efficacy. The first progestogen pill was Chlormadinone acetate, which was used in 1969 but withdrawn in 1970. There are six progestogen pills (Table 8.1) which have many advantages over other methods which are often not recognized. Cerazette and Cerelle are newer progestogen-only pills which inhibit ovulation and now offer women a greater choice and a more effective contraceptive.

THE PROGESTOGEN-ONLY PILL

Explanation of the method

The progestogen-only pill (POP) prevents pregnancy in a number of ways. Older progestogen-only pills, such as Micronor, Norgeston, Noriday and Femulen, cause the cervical mucus to thicken, hindering sperm penetrability, and in some cycles it suppresses ovulation; it also renders the endometrium unreceptive for implantation and reduces fallopian tube function. Cerazette and Cerelle cause inhibition of ovulation close to 100 per cent in contrast to other progestogen-only pills (Organon, 1998).

Efficacy

The effectiveness of the POP is between 96 and 99 per cent effective in preventing pregnancy. Cerazette and Cerelle, at 99.6 per cent, are the most effective POPs, as their chief action is inhibition of ovulation unlike the other progestogen-only pills. If used consistently and correctly the efficacy will be higher, but for typical use the efficacy will be lower; this may be due to women not taking their pills on time (referred to as user error).

Research has shown (Vessey *et al.*, 1985, 1990) that if a woman is heavier than 70kg there is a trend to indicate that the failure rate is higher; however, the numbers were too small in this study to be conclusive. The Clinical Effectiveness Unit

(FSRH, 2008d) states that there is no evidence to support taking two traditional progestogen-only pills a day. Cerazette and Cerelle's efficacy has been shown not to be affected by weight and, as they are the most effective progestogen-only pills, they should be considered first.

Disadvantages

- To be effective, it needs to be taken correctly.
- Irregular menstrual cycle.
- A small number of women develop functional ovarian cysts.
- If POP fails, it may lead to a possible increased ectopic pregnancy rate.
- Effect of POP on breast cancer (see discussion below).

Advantages

- Does not inhibit lactation, so suitable for breast-feeding mothers (this includes Cerazette).
- No evidence of increased risk of cardiovascular disease.
- No evidence of increased risk of venous thromboembolism.
- No evidence of increased risk of hypertension.
- Does not need to be stopped prior to surgery.
- Suitable for women with diabetes or focal migraines.
- Reduction in dysmenorrhoea.
- May relieve premenstrual symptoms.
- Suitable for women unable to take oestrogen.

UKMEC 4 unacceptable health risk: absolute contra-indication

- Current breast cancer.
- Pregnancy.
- Allergy to a constituent.

UKMEC 3 risks outweigh the benefits of using method: relative contra-indication

- History of breast cancer in the past five years.
- Current history of ischaemic heart disease, including cerebrovascular accident, and transient ischaemic attack while taking progestogen methods needs to be reviewed.
- Recent gestational trophoblastic disease.
- Present liver disease, liver adenoma or cancer.
- Positive or unknown Antiphospholipid antibodies.
- Drugs which interfere with the efficacy of the POP (e.g. enzyme-inducing drugs).
- Undiagnosed genital tract bleeding should be investigated.
- Acute porphyrias.

Range of method

The progestogen-only pill contains the same amount of progestogen throughout the packet and is taken every day. Of the six available progestogen pills, three are made from or convert to the progestogen Norethisterone, and one is made from the progestogen Levonorgestrel (Table 8.1). Cerazette and Cerelle are made from the progestogen Desogestrel.

Decision of choice

The introduction of Cerazette and Cerelle, which have a higher contraceptive efficacy and offer a window period of 12 hours compared to traditional progestogen pills, has meant that sometimes prescribers have given cheaper traditional pills whose efficacy is lower because they are cheaper. All clients should be offered the most effective form of progestogen pill currently available, particularly those who are more fertile or clients requiring a high-efficacy contraceptive. Otherwise, as no research has found any difference in efficacy between the Norethisterone and Levonorgestrel traditional progestogen preparations, the most suitable choice between them is the one that gives your client fewer side effects and less irregular bleeding. However, Microval and Norgeston are the most suitable for women breast-feeding, as only tiny amounts of progestogen are found in breast milk with these pills (Guillebaud, 1999). Although Cerazette inhibits ovulation, lactation is not affected (Bjarnadottir *et al.*, 2001).

With the introduction of Cerazette, there has been new research on progestogen-only pills. Two studies comparing Cerazette to Levonorgestrel preparations (Rice *et al.*, 1999; Collaborative Study Group, 1998) have shown Cerazette to have a significant inhibition of ovulation. Cerazette users had a higher incidence of amenorrhoea and infrequent bleeding, although some users experienced frequent bleeding and prolonged bleeding at the beginning of the study.

There have been concerns about Depoprovera, the injectable method, and osteoporosis; however, there are no concerns about other progestogen methods, although the data are limited. If a woman is a long-term user of the progestogen-only pill and has amenorrhoea and complains of hot flushes and vaginal dryness, she should be investigated to see if she is menopausal.

Research on lipid metabolism and the POP shows that there is a negligible effect (McCann and Potter, 1994). However, there may be a decrease in HDL and

Table 8.1 Progestogen-only pills

Pill type	Preparation	Manufacturer	Micrograms per pill	Type of progestogen
Micronor	28-day pill	Janssen	350mcg	Norethisterone
Noriday	28-day pill	Searle	350mcg	Norethisterone
Femulen	28-day pill	Pharmacia	500mcg	Ethynodiol diacetate*
Norgeston	35-day pill	Bayer	30mcg	Levonorgestrel
Cerazette	28-day pill	Organon	75mcg	Desogestrel
Cerelle	28-day pill	Consilient Health	75mcg	Desogestrel

Note
* Converted (>90%) to Norethisterone as the active metabolite.

HDL2 cholesterol. Progestogen pills may be appropriate for women with lipid abnormalities, but this will depend on the severity, and close monitoring will need to be performed.

Breast cancer is a hormone-dependent cancer, so taking any hormones may worsen current or recent breast cancer (FSRH, 2009a). There is no definitive research on the combined pill or progestogen methods; however, going on the worst case scenario the 1996 Collaborative Group on Hormonal Factors in Breast Cancer (Collaborative Group, 1996b) found that the risk of breast cancer was similar to that of the combined pill, while other studies have shown no increased risk. The risk of breast cancer should be lower with progestogen methods than the combined pill, as there is no oestrogen in it. However, any risk is likely to be small, but this is an area where the evidence is unclear. All women should be encouraged to practise breast self-awareness and seek advice early from their general practitioner if they find any changes in their breasts.

Side effects

- Functional ovarian cysts.
- Breast tenderness.
- Bloatedness.
- Depression.
- Fluctuations in weight.
- Nausea.
- Irregular bleeding.
- Amenorrhoea.

How to take the POP

The progestogen pill should be commenced on the first day of a woman's menstrual period with no extra precautions required. The POP is taken every day with no break. If your client needs to change to another progestogen pill then the first pill of the new packet should be commenced the next day with no break; in this case no additional contraception will be required. Broad spectrum antibiotics do not reduce the efficacy of the POP so no extra precautions are required while taking them.

If the progestogen-only pill is commenced following a full-term pregnancy then it should be started from day 21 after birth; no additional precautions are required. If your client has had a miscarriage or termination of pregnancy the POP should be commenced the same day or the following day with no additional precautions required.

Loss of efficacy through drug interaction

Enzyme-inducing drugs (see Table 8.2) reduce the efficacy of the POP, so another form of contraception should be discussed (e.g. the Depoprovera injectable given at intervals of 12 weeks is preferable or condoms should be used while taking the drug and for four weeks after the enzyme-inducing drug has been ceased).

Table 8.2 Enzyme-inducing drugs which reduce the efficacy of the POP

Drug type	Drug
Anticonvulsants	Carbamazepine
	Esilcarbazepine
	Oxcarbazepine
	Phenytoin
	Perampanel
	Phenobarbital
	Primidone
	Topiramate
	Rifinamide
Antitubercle	Rifamycins (e.g. Rifampicin, Rifabutin)
Antiretroviral: Protease inhibitors	Ritonavir
	Ritonavir boosted atazanavir
	Ritonavir boosted tipranavir
	Ritonavir boosted saquinavir
	Nelfinaavir, Darunavir, Fosamprenavir, Lopinavir
Antiretroviral: Non-nucleoside reverse transcriptase inhibitors	Nevirapine
	Efavirenz
Other enzyme-inducing drugs	Modafinil
	Bosentan
	Aprepitant
	Sugammadex
Homeopathic	St Johns Wort

Missed pill rules

If your client takes Cerazette or Cerelle 12 or more hours late she will need to take her pill as soon as she remembers and use extra precautions for two days. For all other traditional progestogen pills, if your client takes her pill three or more hours late she should be advised to take her pill when she remembers and use additional contraceptive precautions for the next two days. If a woman has severe diarrhoea or vomits within two hours of taking any progestogen pill and fails to take another she will need to use extra precautions while having diarrhoea and vomiting and for two days afterwards.

Initial consultation

When counselling a client initially about the progestogen-only pill it is important to explain how this method prevents pregnancy and discuss its efficacy; this will help her understand why it is necessary to take this type of pill on time. A full past and present medical history should be taken, including a family history. If a client has a family history of heart disease then appropriate screening for lipids should be performed. Routine screening of blood pressure, weight and height will indicate whether a client is 70kg or more in weight. If the client is over 70kg in weight, Cerazette is the most effective progestogen-only pill. Details about the last menstrual period are important and a pregnancy test may need to be performed to exclude pregnancy.

Initial counselling should cover breast awareness, safer sex and cervical cytology history as well as emergency contraception. If there is any evidence of cervical, uterine or pelvic infection then screening and treatment should be undertaken. If a cervical smear is due this should be discussed with the client. It may be more appropriate to perform this at the next visit in three months' time. The progestogen pill will not protect against sexually transmitted diseases or HIV and this issue should be discussed sensitively with the client. Many clients choose to use condoms with the progestogen pill to increase its efficacy; however, sometimes men and women fail to think about safer sex.

You should discuss how to take the progestogen pill and when to use extra precautions. Side effects may be experienced initially and you should warn your client that breast tenderness, bloatedness, depression, fluctuations in weight, nausea and irregular bleeding may be experienced. These usually improve with time, so it is important that your client continues with the pill because changing pills may perpetuate the problem. Your client may suffer irregular bleeding which may improve, but pathology should be excluded first. Screening for infection and cervical cytology should be performed along with a bimanual examination. She may also experience amenorrhoea, which may be due to the POP suppressing ovulation. However, if there is any likelihood of pregnancy this should be excluded. Given time your client may wish to discuss sexual anxieties, but sometimes clients leave this to the next visit when they know you better. Always give them the opportunity to bring up the subject by asking open-ended questions like 'Is there anything else you want to discuss?'

Up-to-date leaflets should be given so that your client can refer to them in an emergency along with relevant telephone numbers. Initially a woman is prescribed three months' supply of the progestogen pill and given an appointment for this time.

The points to be covered at the initial consultation are summarized in Box 8.1.

BOX 8.1

Points to be covered at initial consultation

- Full past and present medical history, including family history.
- Record blood pressure, weight, height.
- Details of last menstrual period.
- Discuss efficacy of POP.
- Teach how to take the pill and when to use extra precautions.
- Discuss emergency contraception, safer sex, cervical cytology and breast awareness.
- Discuss side effects.
- Give appropriate leaflets and contact numbers.

Subsequent visits

When a woman initially commences the POP she will return for a follow-up visit in three months' time. If there are no problems she should be seen every six months after this initial follow-up. Discuss with her how she feels about the progestogen pill. Has she taken it on time? Has she had any problems with her pill and what are they? Is she getting a regular menstrual cycle? If her menstrual cycle has been irregular or she has experienced amenorrhoea, is this due to failure to take her pill on time or is there risk of pregnancy? A pregnancy test may need to be performed to exclude this possibility.

Routine observations for blood pressure and weight should be performed. You may find that your client is more relaxed at this visit and may wish to discuss sexual problems or anxieties. This is also a good opportunity to discuss and perform cervical smears if due. You may need to revise how to take the progestogen pill, as clients have to absorb a great deal of information at initial visits and may forget or be confused about missed pill rules.

If there are no problems a six-month supply of the progestogen pill may be prescribed with a supply of condoms if required.

The points to be covered at subsequent visits are summarized in Box 8.2.

BOX 8.2

Points to be covered at subsequent visits

- Update of medical and family history.
- Basic observations: BP, weight, height.
- Date of last menstrual period, has she had any problems with her pill?
- Is her cervical smear due?
- Is she breast aware?
- Do missed pill rules need revision?
- Safer sex: is she at risk?
- Has she got up-to-date leaflets on the POP and emergency contraception?
- Have relevant telephone numbers for advice been given?

SELF-ASSESSMENT QUESTIONS

Answers and discussion at the end of the chapter.

1   What problems would you envisage a woman may encounter on the POP?
2   How would you solve these problems?
3   Which women are most suitable for the POP?
4   Which women are least suitable for the POP?

PROBLEMS ENCOUNTERED

No menstrual period

As long as pregnancy has been excluded you can reassure your client that her pill is working very effectively and preventing ovulation and periods.

Irregular bleeding

Check that your client is taking her pills correctly and not taking them late, which may put her at risk of pregnancy. Ask her to keep a diary of her bleeding pattern so that you can review this at the next visit. You should perform a pregnancy test and STI screen to eliminate the possibility that she is pregnant or has a sexually transmitted infection, as these may cause irregular bleeding too. She may need to change to a different type of progestogen pill, or a different method.

Complaints of nausea

Check that she is not taking her pill on an empty stomach. If the problem continues, change to a different progestogen.

Breast tenderness

Examine breasts. Taking evening primrose oil can help to ease breast tenderness. Changing to a different progestogen may help.

Problems remembering pills

If a woman is frequently forgetting to take her pill this will affect the efficacy of the progestogen pill and put her at risk of pregnancy. Check what time she is taking her pill, and whether there is a more convenient time to take it. Can she set an alarm on her watch or computer diary, or put a reminder on her mobile phone? What about carrying her packet around with her? Discuss with her how she feels about forgetting her pill. Would another method of contraception be more suitable?

SEXUALITY AND ANXIETIES

The progestogen pill may not always be a woman's first choice of contraception. She may have initially requested the combined pill but has a contra-indication to it. This may affect compliance and increase dissatisfaction with the progestogen pill.

CASE STUDY 8.1

A 24-year-old woman consults requesting to start the pill. She is aware of other methods but feels pills would suit her best. The combined pill and the progestogen pill are discussed, and the risks, disadvantages and advantages are fully covered. The client summarizes the counselling by saying that the combined pill will involve regular periods but carries a risk of venous thromboembolism, while the progestogen pill, Cerazette, has the same effectiveness in preventing pregnancy and has fewer risks but irregular bleeding. She decides on this information to try the progestogen pill Cerazette as it has fewer risks, and to 'put up' with the irregular bleeding.

Many women hold the misconception that the progestogen pill is ineffective because it was called the 'mini-pill', which may stop women from choosing it. However, it is a safe, reliable and effective method if taken consistently by the client.

Women who fail to take their pill on time may subconsciously wish to become pregnant but may not be ready to admit this to themselves. Given time and sensitive counselling they may feel able to discuss this issue.

ANSWERS TO SELF-ASSESSMENT QUESTIONS

1   *What problems would you envisage a woman may encounter on the POP?*

Women may complain of premenstrual-like symptoms such as breast tenderness, nausea, irregular bleeding or amenorrhoea. They may find it difficult to remember when to take their pill, and if they have taken the combined pill previously they may dislike the lack of warning about their menstrual cycle.

2   *How would you solve these problems?*

Nausea can be solved by always taking the pill after food. Premenstrual-like symptoms may be reduced by trying evening primrose oil and vitamin B6. If there is no improvement then changing to a different POP may help.

Problems with irregular bleeding and amenorrhoea should be discussed. Often if women are fully counselled on how the POP works in preventing pregnancy they are more ready to accept any problems. Check they are taking their pills correctly and whether they understand the importance of this in relation to efficacy.

3   *Which women are most suitable for the POP?*

Women who are most suitable to take the POP are those who are breast-feeding and those who are older. It is also suitable for diabetic women, or for women undergoing surgery, or women who suffer migraines or have had a venous thromboembolism or who smoke – all of whom are unable to take the combined pill. There are in fact very few women who are not suitable for this method.

4   *Which women are least suitable for the POP?*

Women who are less suitable to take the POP are women who are unreliable about taking pills or who find the irregular bleeding a problem. It is not suitable for women who are taking liver enzyme-inducing drugs where there will be loss of efficacy. It is not suitable for women who are pregnant. Women who have had an ectopic pregnancy, or who have been hospitalized with functional ovarian cysts should be given Cerazette or Cerelle, as this will inhibit ovulation and reduce the risk of functional ovarian cysts and ectopic pregnancy.

Any woman who has experienced a problem with the combined pill which may not be related to the oestrogen content of the COC or who has had a malignancy of the breast should not be given the POP. It should not be given to women who suffer any liver disease or arterial disease, or who are taking any drugs which may reduce the efficacy of the POP. Table 8.2 outlines enzyme-inducing drugs which reduce the efficacy of the POP through the induction of liver enzymes, which increase the metabolism of the progestogen pill.

INJECTABLE CONTRACEPTION

- Introduction and history
- The injectable method of contraception
- Sexuality and anxieties

INTRODUCTION AND HISTORY

Injectables were initially a result of research following the war, when Dr Junkman found in 1953 that a long-acting injection was created if progestogen and alcohol were combined.

In 1957 research began on the injectable Norigest, now known as Noristerat, which is licensed for short-term use in the UK, i.e. following administration of the rubella vaccine. In 1963 trials commenced on the injectable Depoprovera, which was licensed in the UK for long-term use in 1984 when other methods were not suitable. Since 1990 it has been licensed as a first-choice method.

Of the two injectables available, Depoprovera is the most widely used. However, many women are still unaware of its existence or are given inaccurate information, hindering its acceptance as a method.

THE INJECTABLE METHOD OF CONTRACEPTION

Explanation of the method

Like the progestogen pill, injectables prevent pregnancy in a number of ways. They cause the cervical mucus to thicken, thus stopping sperm penetrability, render the endometrium unreceptive for implantation, and reduce fallopian tube function. However, the main function of injectables in preventing pregnancy is the suppression of ovulation.

Efficacy

The efficacy of injectables is between 99 and 100 per cent in preventing pregnancy. Research has shown that Depoprovera, if given at least every 12 weeks, has a failure rate of fewer than 4 in 1000 over two years (FSRH, 2008b). Injectables are a highly effective form of contraception as user failure rates are reduced. This is because women do not have to remember to take a pill and there is no loss of efficacy caused by diarrhoea and vomiting.

Disadvantages

- Irregular bleeding or spotting, or amenorrhoea.
- Delay in return of fertility of up to a year.
- Depression.
- Weight gain.
- Galactorrhoea.
- Once given cannot be withdrawn.
- May have an association with osteoporosis with long-term use.
- Effect of injectables on breast cancer (see p. 92).

Advantages

- High efficacy.
- Lasts 8 to 12 weeks.
- Reduction in dysmenorrhoea and menorrhagia resulting in less anaemia.
- Reduction in premenstrual symptoms.
- Less pelvic inflammatory disease.
- Possible reduction of endometriosis owing to thickened cervical mucus.
- Efficacy not reduced by diarrhoea, vomiting or antibiotics.

UKMEC 4 unacceptable health risk: absolute contra-indication

- Current breast cancer.
- Pregnancy.
- Allergy to a constituent.
- Acute porphyrias.
- Current osteoporosis, osteopenia.

UKMEC 3 risks outweigh the benefits of using method: relative contra-indication

- Multiple risk factors for cardiovascular disease.
- History of breast cancer in the past five years.
- Current history of ischaemic heart disease, including cerebrovascular accident and transient ischaemic attack while taking progestogen methods needs to be reviewed.
- Risk factors for osteoporosis.
- Recent gestational trophoblastic disease.
- Present liver disease, liver adenoma or cancer.
- Positive or unknown Antiphospholipid antibodies.
- Severe thrombocyopenia.
- Diabetes with retinopathy/neuropathy or vascular disease.
- Drugs which interfere with the efficacy of the POP (e.g. enzyme-inducing drugs).
- Undiagnosed genital tract bleeding should be investigated.

Range of method

There are two types of injectables: Depoprovera and Noristerat.

Depoprovera

Depoprovera (abbreviated to DMPA) contains depot medroxyprogesterone acetate and is given in a single 150mg injection deep intramuscularly every 12 weeks. It is now available in a pre-filled syringe and licensed to be given no later than 12 weeks and 5 days after the last injection.

Noristerat

Noristerat (abbreviated to NET EN) contains norethisterone oenanthate and is given in a single 200mg injection intramuscularly every eight weeks.

Decision of choice

Noristerat is licensed for short-term use only; this means that no more than two consecutive injections may be given. Noristerat is usually used as a method following vasectomy or rubella administration where a highly effective method is required for a short period of time.

Depoprovera is licensed for long-term use. It is suitable for most women, particularly those who forget their pills, and for women on the COC taking drugs where there is a loss of efficacy. However, there is a lack of information about long-term amenorrhoea, which is usually a result of this injection, and its implications. In 1991 research (Cundy *et al.*, 1991) suggested that women who are using long-term Depoprovera may be partially oestrogen deficient; this may have an adverse effect on bone density and may give an increased risk of osteoporosis. However, Cundy *et al.* (1994) showed that this effect may be completely reversible once oestrogen levels have returned to normal following cessation of Depoprovera. The CSAC advises (CSAC, 1993a) that following five years of amenorrhoea a serum oestradiol should be taken. However, Guillebaud (1999) suggests that as oestradiol levels can be low whether a woman is amenorrhoeic or not it is important to ascertain if she is suffering from symptoms of hypo-oestrogenism such as vaginal dryness, loss of libido and hot flushes. If she is experiencing symptoms or is a smoker, she should be screened or change method; if, however, she is a non-smoker and symptom-free, after discussion she may defer screening. If the serum oestradiol is less than 100pmol I^{-1} this indicates oestrogen deficiency. Additional oestrogen would be appropriate and another method of contraception may be more suitable. Bone density screening may be indicated along with close supervision of the situation. However, a definitive evidence-based guideline for management of women using Depoprovera long term is unavailable due to conflicting studies. Gbolade (2002) states that loss of bone density in long-term users appears to be transient and reversible; however, it is important that women are counselled about the possible long-term risk. A recent study (Ryan *et al.*, 2002) formed the view that women with risk factors for osteoporosis should be screened for bone densitometry prior to commencement. Risk factors for osteoporosis include personal history of fractures or anorexia nervosa, being an amenorrhoeic athlete, smoking, family history of osteoporosis in a first-degree relative, and use of steroids including oral steroids. Careful history taking to highlight these risks is important. In addition, it is good practice to encourage women to maintain and build skeletal mass through diet, exercise and avoidance of smoking and alcohol.

The World Health Organization has categorized Depoprovera as category 2 for young women under the age of 18 rather than category 1 (always usable) because of concerns over bone density. Category 2 means that the method is broadly usable where the benefits outweigh the risks (FSRH, 2009a). Bone density is still being established in under-16s following commencement of menarche. For many young women this may be the most suitable method if they are unable to take the combined pill and are at risk of pregnancy. The Clinical Effectiveness Unit advises that women over 45 years can continue with progestogen-only injectable contraception up until the maximum age of 50 as long as they are reviewed every two years to assess potential risks (FSRH, 2010c).

The risk factors for breast cancer for the injectable contraceptive were found to be similar to those of the combined pill (see p. 92).

There is no increased risk of cervical (International Family Planning Perspectives, 1992; WHO, 1992) or ovarian cancer with the use of Depoprovera; however, there is a protective effect for endometrial cancer (Pisake, 1994).

When counselling women about the risk of osteoporosis and breast cancer in relation to injectables, please note that much of the research to date is inconclusive. Hopefully studies currently underway will help resolve this dilemma.

Side effects

- Headaches.
- Bloatedness.
- Depression.
- Weight gain.
- Mood swings.
- Irregular bleeding.
- Amenorrhoea.

How to give injectables

Ideally, Depoprovera should be given within the first five days of a menstrual period; no additional contraception is required. After this, injections should be given every 12 weeks.

Noristerat should be given on the first day of the menstrual period; no additional contraception is required. After this injections should be given every eight weeks.

Injections should be given deep intramuscularly into the upper outer quadrant of the buttock. The Depoprovera pre-filled syringe should be shaken well before being given. The Noristerat ampoule should be warmed to body temperature before being given. This will make it easier to draw up, as it is mixed with castor oil. Injection sites should not be massaged after administration of the injectable as this will reduce its efficacy.

Following first-trimester termination of pregnancy and miscarriage the first injection is usually given within the first five days with no extra precautions required. Post-partum women should commence their first injectable five to six weeks following delivery, since if it is given earlier there is increased and prolonged menstrual bleeding.

Loss of efficacy through drug interaction

There is no loss of efficacy with Depoprovera or Noristerat with broad spectrum antibiotics and enzyme-inducing drugs. The injections should continue to be given at 12 weeks and 5 days for Depoprovera and 8 weeks for Noristerat (FSRH, 2011b).

SELF-ASSESSMENT QUESTIONS

Answers and discussion at the end of the chapter.

1 Who would you consider most suitable for using Depoprovera as a method of contraception?
2 What would you do if a woman was beyond 12 weeks for her next Depoprovera injection?
3 Name five issues that should be covered during counselling for women considering the Depoprovera injection.

Initial consultation

Women who consult who are interested in choosing Depoprovera as a form of contraception should be counselled carefully, as this is a less easily reversed method. Counselling should cover the following areas to enable the woman to make an informed decision:

1 Once injected it cannot be removed. It is important that women accept that once given, the injection cannot be withdrawn, so any unwanted side effects they experience, although usually short-lived, will continue until the injection expires at 12 weeks.
2 Efficacy and frequency of injections. Counselling should involve efficacy and how frequently injections need to be given. Occasionally women have been under the impression that Depoprovera is given every three months. This can be longer than 12 weeks, so it is important to talk about frequency of intervals in weeks. If a client is due a holiday, for example, her injection can be given earlier.
3 Menstrual disturbances. Women should be warned that they may experience irregular bleeding initially with Depoprovera or amenorrhoea within the first year. If warned beforehand women usually find this acceptable.
4 Return of fertility. There can be a delay in the return of periods and fertility; however, most women will become pregnant within one year of stopping Depoprovera. There is no evidence that Depoprovera causes permanent

infertility. If a woman is thinking of becoming pregnant in the near future then another form of contraception may be more appropriate.

5 Weight gain and other minor side effects. There may be a small weight gain, so if women are aware of this they will be able to monitor it and it may be avoided.

6 Depression may be experienced by some women, although this may be due to outside factors.

7 Long-term use and the possible risk of osteoporosis are at present being researched. Clients often ask about the long-term effects of amenorrhoea, and as new information comes to light they should be informed.

Women may wish to be given time before commencing injectables to think about their decision. Timing of the initial injection should be discussed along with alternative contraception. The first injection should be administered within the first five days of the cycle; otherwise contraceptive precautions will be required for seven days. If there has been any unprotected sexual intercourse or there is any concern over pregnancy then a pregnancy test and bimanual examination if appropriate may need to be performed to exclude pregnancy.

Routine observations of weight, height and blood pressure should be monitored. A full medical history of the woman and family should be obtained. Previous contraceptive history should be discussed. If she has used a progestogen method previously this will give an impression of how she will experience the injectable. A cervical smear may need to be performed if due, although this may have to be deferred until the next injection if it is during her menses or if she prefers. Injectables do not protect against sexually transmitted diseases and HIV, so issues around safer sex may need to be discussed and approached with the woman.

Up-to-date literature about the injectable should be given, along with an appointment for when the next injection will be due.

The points to be covered at the initial consultation are summarized in Box 9.1.

BOX 9.1

Points to be covered at initial consultation

- Full past and present medical history, including family history.
- Record BP, weight, height.
- Details of last menstrual period and any unprotected sexual intercourse.
- Discuss efficacy of injectable.
- Discuss intervals when injectables should be given.
- Discuss emergency contraception, safer sex, cervical cytology and breast awareness.
- Discuss side effects and issues around Depoprovera (nos 1–7 above).
- Give appropriate leaflets and contact numbers.

Subsequent visits

Subsequent injections of Depoprovera should be given every 12 weeks and Noristerat at 8-week intervals. Observations of blood pressure and weight should be performed. Regular weight checks can be useful as often clients complain that their weight has increased, yet when they are weighed there is no change.

At subsequent consultations it is important to find out how your client is finding her injection. Is she experiencing any problems? How can these be alleviated? (See 'Problems encountered'). Most side effects of injectables are short-lived (e.g. breakthrough bleeding), so it is worth persevering with this method.

BOX 9.2

Points to be covered at subsequent visits

- Update of medical and family history.
- Basic observations: BP, weight.
- Has she had any problems (e.g. bleeding)?
- Is her cervical smear due?
- Is she breast aware?
- Safer sex: is she at risk?
- Has she got up-to-date leaflets on the injectable?
- Have relevant telephone numbers for advice been given?

It is important that your client knows when her next injection is due, and that she keeps a record of the date of her previous injection in case she has to attend another nurse or doctor for her injection.

PROBLEMS ENCOUNTERED

Irregular bleeding pattern

If a woman suffers irregular bleeding she should be advised to return before her next injection is due, so that it can be given earlier. If there is no improvement in the bleeding pattern then she may be prescribed concurrent oestrogen either by the combined pill or, if this is contra-indicated, by hormone replacement therapy.

Most women who experience breakthrough bleeding find that this usually resolves by the fourth injection.

Complaints of increased acne and mood swings

Some women may complain of increased acne or mood swings. This usually improves, but vitamin B6 and evening primrose oil may be beneficial. If there is no improvement in symptoms, this should be discussed with the woman. She may wish to change method or treat the acne, for example, if she has a limited choice of contraception.

Clients attending late for injections

Women who regularly attend late for their injections may need help with reminders. Some family planning clinics run domiciliary services for this reason, or send their clients reminders. Try making your client's next appointment earlier at 12-week intervals.

If your client is beyond 12 weeks and 5 days since her last injection of Depoprovera then you may give it up to 14 weeks (or up to 10 weeks if Noristerat) since the last injection with no extra precautions or emergency contraception required. If she is beyond 14 weeks and 1 day since her last Depoprovera or 10 weeks and 1 day since her last Noristerat and there has been no unprotected sexual intercourse then you can give the Depoprovera or Noristerat with extra precautions required for 7 days and a pregnancy test is recommended in 21 days. If there has been unprotected sexual intercourse and this has happened in the past 5 days, emergency contraception – either hormonal or a PCIUD – will be required and the injection may be given with extra precautions taken for 7 days (or if EllaOne is given extra precautions will be required for 14 days) (FSRH, 2010a) and a pregnancy test performed in 21 days.

If the last injection was more than 14 weeks and 1 day ago (or Noristerat 10 weeks and one day) and there has been unprotected sex over 5 days ago, then you are unable to give emergency contraception and you should advise alternative contraception or no sexual intercourse and perform a pregnancy test in 21 days.

This is outside the drug licence but is recommended practice by the Faculty of Sexual and Reproductive Healthcare (FSRH, 2008b) (see Box 9.3).

SEXUALITY AND ANXIETIES

Injectables are a highly effective form of contraception. They give a great deal of freedom to a woman, only requiring a consultation every 8 to 12 weeks. They allow women time to think and delay decisions about permanent methods of contraception. However, they are not a widely used method. Many women hold misconceptions about the injectable which may also be held by professionals. Fears that the injection causes permanent infertility and foetal abnormality have been researched (Wilson, 1993). Although no evidence has been found to support these anxieties, they still remain. In the meantime injectables are in many instances undervalued and many women are not even informed of the availability of this method.

Many women feel that having an injection which causes amenorrhoea is unnatural. There is concern about menstrual loss – 'Where does it all go?' 'Doesn't all the blood build up?' – which emphasizes the need to explain clearly how the reproductive cycle works and how it is affected by the injectable. Women often forget that during pregnancy and while breast-feeding there is little or no bleeding, and this is natural. However, for some women the experience of amenorrhoea can be too worrying. A period is the way women normally know whether they are pregnant or not, and can be very reassuring.

BOX 9.3

What to do if a Depoprovera injection is late?

This practice would be unlicensed so would be off label but is endorsed by the Clinical Effective Unit for the Faculty of Sexual and Reproductive Healthcare (FSRH, 2008b).

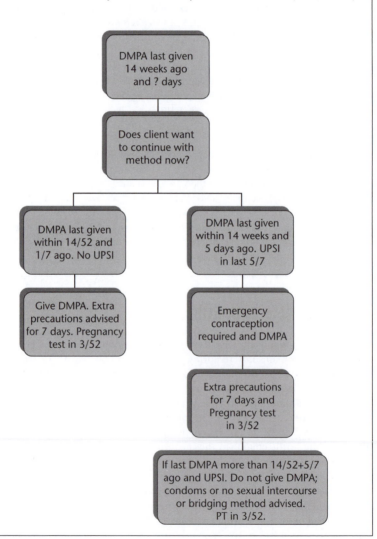

ANSWERS TO SELF-ASSESSMENT QUESTIONS

1 *Who would you consider most suitable for using Depoprovera as a method of contraception?*

Women who are most suitable for using Depoprovera are:

- Women who do not want to become pregnant but are not yet ready to choose sterilization, or do not wish to become pregnant in the foreseeable future.
- Women who are having treatment with liver enzyme-inducing drugs (e.g. Rifampicin for tuberculosis).
- Women who are unable to take the combined pill.
- Young women who want a highly effective form of contraception, but either do not want to take the COC or have an absolute contra-indication to it, or find it difficult to remember to take it.

2 *What would you do if a woman was beyond 12 weeks for her next Depoprovera injection?*

If your client has gone beyond 12 weeks and 5 days then you can give the next injection as long as it is within 14 weeks with no need for emergency contraception or extra precautions required. If it is more than 14 weeks and 1 day since the last injection, refer to Box 9.3.

3 *Name five issues that should be covered during counselling for women considering the Depoprovera injection.*

Five issues that should be discussed during counselling include the following:

- Efficacy.
- Delay in return of fertility.
- Amenorrhoea and irregular bleeding pattern.
- Once given, the injection cannot be withdrawn.
- Side effects (e.g. weight gain, depression and long-term effects of injectables which are uncertain, like research into osteoporosis).

10 CONTRACEPTIVE IMPLANTS

■ Introduction and history
■ Nexplanon
■ The future
■ Sexuality and anxieties

INTRODUCTION AND HISTORY

In 1966 The Population Council commenced research into implants, which showed that silastic rubber capsules released continuous levels of steroid hormone for more than a year. In 1975 the first long-term trial was initiated with six elastomer capsules called Norplant. In May 1993 Norplant was approved for use in the UK as a contraceptive. Norplant was licensed for five years and is no longer manufactured. Norplant received a great deal of adverse media attention after some women had problems with insertion and removal of the capsules; as a result Implanon was launched, although many women were very happy with Norplant. Implanon was a single capsule, reducing problems with insertion and removal. However, while Implanon was easier to fit and remove, the insertion procedure was slightly complicated and the manufacturers addressed this by developing Nexplanon in 2010. Nexplanon and Implanon are the same implants; however, the applicator and insertion technique for Nexplanon is more straightforward to ensure correct placement of the capsule. Nexplanon is now the only licensed implant in the UK. Nexplanon should always be inserted by professionals who have undergone the designated training for this device to avoid problems with incorrect insertion and, as a result, difficulties with removal.

NEXPLANON

Nexplanon is a single rod which contains 68mg of etonogestrel, a metabolite of the progestogen Desogestrel, which is inserted subdermally and licensed for three years. The rod is 4cm with a diameter of 2mm and is provided with a sterile pre-loaded applicator, and is radiopaque. Nexplanon prevents pregnancy by inhibiting ovulation, mucus and endometrial effect.

Efficacy

There have been no pregnancies in the clinical trials to date (Edwards and Moore, 1999). Nexplanon has the advantage of having a high efficacy because it has a no user failure rate – there is no need to remember to take a pill or insert a diaphragm.

Norplant studies have shown that for women who weigh more than 70kg the gross cumulative five-year pregnancy rate is slightly higher than for lighter women (Sivin, 1988). There have been concerns that contraceptive efficacy for this group may be reduced with Nexplanon. However, further research has shown that there have been no pregnancies, and, as a result, contraceptive efficacy is not reduced in women with a BMI over 30kg m^{-2} (FSRH, 2008c).

Disadvantages

- Requires a trained professional to insert and remove implants.
- Irregular menstrual bleeding such as amenorrhoea, spotting.
- Minor side effects such as headaches, acne, etc.
- Possible discomfort or infection at site.

Advantages

- High efficacy.
- Easily reversed.
- Long-term contraception.
- Free from oestrogen side effects.
- Low user failure: once in place there is nothing to remember.

UKMEC 4 unacceptable health risk: absolute contra-indication

- Current breast cancer.
- Pregnancy.
- Allergy to components of implant.

UKMEC 3 risks outweigh the benefits of using method: relative contra-indication

- Undiagnosed genital tract bleeding.
- Acute porphyria.
- Current thromboembolic disease.
- Current ischaemic heart disease, cardiovascular accident.
- Active liver disease with moderately abnormal liver function results, gall-bladder disease, viral hepatitis, benign or malignant liver tumours.
- Liver enzyme-inducing drugs.
- Breast cancer in the past five years.

- Sex steroid cancers.
- Positive antiphospholipid disorder.

Range of method

Nexplanon is the only implant available in the UK. It is 4cm in length and 2mm in diameter, and is inserted with a disposable sterile applicator.

Side effects

- Irregular bleeding, amenorrhoea, or frequent and prolonged bleeding.
- Pain, itching or infection at insertion site.
- Headaches.
- Nausea.
- Mood changes.
- Weight changes.
- Acne.

Decision of choice

Women who are at risk of pregnancy or who have become pregnant because they have difficulty remembering to take a contraceptive pill or use another contraceptive method (user failure) may find Nexplanon a useful alternative. Women choosing Nexplanon as their method of contraception should be counselled carefully about side effects, as this will influence their final decision. Nexplanon is suitable for women who have completed or wish to delay starting their family.

Research has shown that 80 per cent of women's menstrual cycles returned to normal or to their pre-trial pattern within three months (Edwards and Moore, 1999), illustrating the reversibility of Nexplanon.

Counselling for Nexplanon

As Nexplanon involves a minor operation it is important to counsel women fully so that they are able to make an informed decision. Women are also more likely to accept and continue with a method if they are aware of any side effects prior to the procedure.

You should discuss with your client the efficacy of Nexplanon, and the procedure for insertion and removal. A full medical history should be taken along with family medical history. Side effects with Nexplanon are similar to any progestogen-only method, so if your client has previously tolerated a progestogen-only method well, this will give you both a good indication on how she will feel with Nexplanon. If your client already suffers from symptoms such as headaches or acne then Nexplanon may not improve these problems. However, many women, if warned, are prepared to accept continuing problems to be assured of a highly effective form of contraception.

Changes in menstrual pattern are the most frequently reported side effect of Nexplanon. Women may experience amenorrhoea, irregular menses or breakthrough bleeding. It is important to discuss the likelihood of amenorrhoea with Nexplanon as this may cause anxiety. Many women find periods very reassuring as they indicate that they are not pregnant, and as a result amenorrhoea can cause great anxiety.

Amenorrhoea occurs in 20 per cent of women, whilst 50 per cent of women will have irregular bleeding which could be prolonged and frequent for six months (FSRH, 2008c). There was no consistent pattern in the bleeding patterns reported in research on implants; if a woman had had amenorrhoea she could still experience irregular bleeding, or vice versa (Edwards and Moore, 1999). Research on clinical experience with Norplant has shown that if women are given careful counselling about Norplant's effects on menstruation there is a higher continuation rate with this method (Mascarenhas *et al.*, 1994), and the same could be said for all methods of contraception.

Following counselling, written up-to-date information should be given, so that your client is able to make an informed decision about Nexplanon.

It is important that your client uses contraception up until the time of Nexplanon insertion to exclude any possibility of pregnancy. Preferably, Nexplanon should be inserted on the first day of your client's menstrual period, where no extra precautions will be required. If Nexplanon is inserted at any other time in the cycle then pregnancy should be excluded first, and additional contraception should be used for seven days following insertion.

Following a termination of pregnancy Nexplanon may be inserted immediately; if inserted later, additional contraception will be required for seven days. After childbirth Nexplanon may be inserted on day 21; if inserted later then extra contraceptive precautions will be required for seven days.

The areas to be covered at counselling are summarized in Box 10.1.

BOX 10.1

Areas to be covered at counselling

- Full medical history.
- Check blood pressure, weight and height.
- Ensure client has contraceptive cover up until and after insertion if needed.
- Take details of last menstrual period; exclude pregnancy if relevant.
- Discuss how Nexplanon works and its efficacy.
- Discuss insertion and removal procedure.
- Discuss side effects.
- Give literature on Nexplanon.
- Organize date for insertion.

Drugs which reduce the efficacy of Nexplanon

Drugs which may reduce the efficacy of Nexplanon are listed in Table 10.1.

Table 10.1 Drugs which reduce the efficacy of Nexplanon

Drug type	Drug
Anticonvulsants	Carbamazepine
	Esilcarbamazepine
	Oxcarbazepine
	Phenytoin
	Perampanel
	Phenobarbital
	Primidone
	Topiramate
	Rifinamide
Antitubercle	Rifamycins (e.g. Rifampicin, Rifabutin)
Antiretroviral: Protease inhibitors	Ritonavir
	Ritonavir boosted atazanavir
	Ritonavir boosted tipranavir
	Ritonavir boosted saquinavir
	Nelfinaavir, Darunavir, Fosamprenavir, Lopinavir
Antiretroviral: Non-nucleoside reverse transcriptase inhibitors	Nevirapine
	Efavirenz
Other enzyme-inducing drugs	Modafinil
	Bosentan
	Aprepitant
	Sugammadex
Homeopathic	St Johns Wort

Loss of efficacy of Nexplanon

Additional barrier contraception is required with Nexplanon if your client is taking liver enzyme-inducing drugs; this is the case both while taking the drugs and for 28 days after their cessation (FSRH, 2011b). Alternatively, a client may be given the injectable contraceptive Depoprovera with no extra precautions required.

Nexplanon insertion

Nexplanon is inserted using a sterile technique under local anaesthetic into the inner aspect of the upper arm of the non-dominant arm (Figs 10.1 to 10.2). Insertion of Nexplanon is performed with a specially designed applicator. Nexplanon should be inserted at the inner side of the upper arm about 8 to 10cm above the medial epicondyle of the humerus. The insertion site should be marked and cleaned with disinfectant, and local anaesthetic given. The skin should be stretched and the tip of the implant applicator inserted into the site at a slight angle of 30 degrees. The capsule is held inside the applicator at the tip. Release the skin and lower the

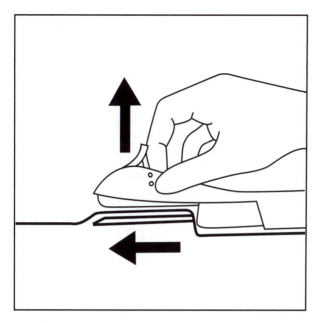

Figure 10.1 Inserting the needle under the skin. (Reproduced with permission of Merck Sharp & Dohme B.V., a subsidiary of Merck & Co. Inc, Whitehouse Stations, New Jersey, USA. All rights reserved)

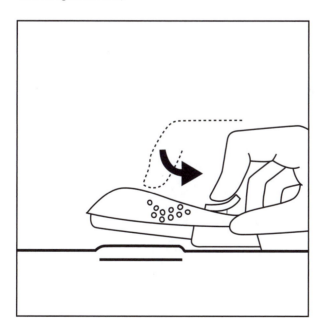

Figure 10.2 Releasing the implant under the skin and removing the applicator. (Reproduced with permission of Merck Sharp & Dohme B.V., a subsidiary of Merck & Co. Inc, Whitehouse Stations, New Jersey, USA. All rights reserved)

applicator to a horizontal position, lift the skin with the tip of the needle but keep the needle in the subdermal connective tissue. While lifting the skin, gently insert the needle to its full length without using force. The purple slider is unlocked by pushing it down slightly and the slider is moved back until it stops; this releases the implant subdermally and locks the needle in the applicator. The applicator is removed and the implant should be palpated. A dry dressing, which should be removed in 5 days, and pressure bandage is applied which may be removed after 24 hours. The insertion procedure takes 15 minutes. Batch number and expiry date of the implant should be recorded in the client's notes.

Women should be able to feel the capsules once *in situ* if they wish to touch the site for reassurance, but they will not be visible unless the woman is very thin. A user card should be given to the client which includes the batch number, date of insertion, the arm where the implant is inserted, name of the inserter, and hospital and intended date of removal.

Subsequent visits

You should see your client three months after insertion to check her insertion site, blood pressure and weight. If she has no problems she should be seen at six-month intervals for monitoring of menstrual cycle, blood pressure and weight. If your client has menstrual irregularities or pain, or swelling around the implant site, she should be advised to return earlier.

Nexplanon removal

Removal of Nexplanon should only be performed by a professional who is familiar with the removal technique. Removal of the implants is performed using a sterile technique with local anaesthetic. The location of the implant should be indicated on the user card, and the location palpated and then marked at the distal end. A non-palpable implant should be located by ultrasound or magnetic resonance imaging (MRI) and removed with the aid of ultrasound.

For removal the area should be cleaned and local anaesthetic inserted under the implant. An incision of 2mm in length is made longitudinally. The implant should be pushed towards the incision until the tip is visible and then be grasped with forceps and removed (Fig. 10.3). The incision site should have a steri-strip applied and sterile dressing and pressure bandage applied.

If your client wishes to continue using Nexplanon as a method of contraception, a new implant may be inserted in a parallel plane from that removed through the same incision. However, if she is discontinuing with this method alternative contraception is required once the capsule is removed.

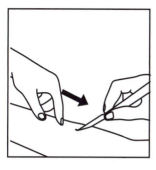

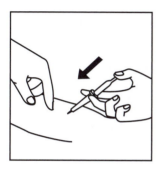
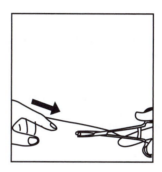

Figure 10.3 Removal of the implant. (Reproduced with permission of Merck Sharp & Dohme B.V., a subsidiary of Merck & Co. Inc, Whitehouse Stations, New Jersey, USA. All rights reserved)

SELF-ASSESSMENT QUESTIONS

Answers and discussion at the end of the chapter.

1   Who do you think is suitable for Nexplanon?
2   What would you do if your client complained of amenorrhoea?
3   How long can Nexplanon remain *in situ*, and when does fertility return?
4   When would you advise your client she would need to commence alternative contraception following removal?

PROBLEMS ENCOUNTERED

Localized skin reactions

Recent research (Blain *et al.*, 1996) has shown that factors which influence localized skin reactions include the use of latex gloves for insertion and removal of the implant, and tension under the first steri-strip applied to the incision.

Irregular bleeding

Research has shown that one of the main reasons for discontinuing Nexplanon is due to complaints of irregular bleeding. Five per cent of women discontinued because of this problem per 6 months in the first 18 months (Edwards and Moore, 1999). This emphasizes the need for comprehensive counselling prior to insertion.

Women who experience persistent irregular bleeding should be screened for sexually transmitted infections, cervical cytology and pregnancy to exclude the possibility of pregnancy or chlamydia/gonorrhoea infection initially. If these tests are negative and the combined pill is not contra-indicated, a three-month supply of a Levonorgestrel-containing pill (second generation) may be given which can be taken continuously or in cyclical regimen. The combined pill is unlicensed for this use but this practice is endorsed by the Faculty of Sexual and Reproductive Healthcare (FSRH, 2009b). If the combined pill is contra-indicated then mefenamic acid can be prescribed at 500mg up to three times a day for five days. These regimens may have a beneficial effect but there are limited data on their success. Women should also be warned that bleeding may return.

Women who experience amenorrhoea with Nexplanon may be alarmed at the loss of their menses if they are not warned prior to insertion. Explaining how Nexplanon prevents pregnancy and why amenorrhoea occurs can help prevent anxiety.

Premenstrual-like symptoms

Women may find that taking evening primrose oil or vitamin B6 will help relieve premenstrual-like symptoms such as irritability and mood swings.

CASE STUDY 10.1

A 26-year-old woman, Jan, has two children aged 2 and 3. She had a miscarriage prior to having her children, and three months previously she had a termination of pregnancy. Jan has requested a sterilization but her current relationship is a new one, and it has been suggested that she should wait a little longer. She is 5'3" (159cm) and weighs 15 stone 2lb (96kg) and was taking the combined pill but has changed to the progestogen pill, which she finds difficult to remember to take on time. Jan has always suffered from painful, heavy periods and all her pregnancies have been unplanned.

The combined pill is contra-indicated in this situation because the BMI is 38kg m^{-2}. Because of Jan's weight the efficacy of the POP may be affected, and she is unsuitable for an IUD because of her dysmenorrhoea and menorrhagia.

On discussion with Jan, three long-term methods of contraception are discussed: the injectable Depoprovera, the implant Nexplanon and the intrauterine system (IUS) Mirena. Jan is reluctant to have the IUS because she does not like the idea of the insertion. She feels that she may not remember to attend for injections every 11 to 12 weeks, leaving Nexplanon as the method of choice. Although she is not keen on the insertion of Nexplanon she prefers this over a Mirena insertion, and decides to go ahead with this as a method of contraception.

THE FUTURE

A two-rod implant called Jadelle is available outside the UK and is licensed for five years; it contains 75mg of Levonorgestrel.

SEXUALITY AND ANXIETIES

Women who choose Nexplanon find its high efficacy and lack of user compliance important advantages. They may be unable to use other methods because of medical contra-indications, or wish to use a method that is long term without making the final permanent decision of sterilization.

Norplant was beset with problems, and misleading information by the media discouraged uptake by women (*The Economist*, 1995; Bromham, 1996). Problems with the removal of Norplant have been widely covered and it has been found that correct placement of the capsules is vital for a problem-free removal procedure. Problems with removal may be because the capsules have been inserted too deeply, making removal difficult. This emphasizes the need to have an appropriately trained professional inserting all implants. The UK distributors of Nexplanon have established a free training programme for doctors to teach insertion and removal techniques to alleviate this problem. The Faculty of Family Planning has introduced a letter of competence in Subdermal Contraceptive Implants for Faculty members for five years from issue and has also developed a regional network of advisers. This has been instigated to validate implant training. Sadly, the media influence women and poor publicity about a method remains in their minds. Many forget the risks of pregnancy and childbirth, and the trauma of a termination of pregnancy.

The introduction of Nexplanon has given women a wider choice of contraception, and offers long-term safety against pregnancy. It gives greater freedom to women who have a limited range of methods to choose from because of medical contra-indications. It is easily reversible once removed, but highly effective when *in situ*.

ANSWERS TO SELF-ASSESSMENT QUESTIONS

1   *Who do you think is suitable for Nexplanon?*

Women who are most suitable for Nexplanon are those who have completed their families, or who do not wish to have children in the near future. Nexplanon is also suitable for women who may be unable to use another method because they have a contra-indication to them (e.g. the combined pill and focal migraines or menorrhagia and the IUD).

2   *What would you do if your client complained of amenorrhoea?*

It is important to exclude pregnancy first. Once this has been excluded you should discuss with your client why amenorrhoea occurs with Nexplanon.

3   *How long can Nexplanon remain* in situ, *and when does fertility return?*

Nexplanon can remain *in situ* for three years. Fertility returns immediately the capsules are removed.

4   *When would you advise your client she would need to commence alternative contraception following removal?*

Another method of contraception should be used immediately Nexplanon is removed.

THE INTRAUTERINE DEVICE (IUD)

11

- Introduction and history
- The intrauterine device
- The future
- Sexuality and anxieties

INTRODUCTION AND HISTORY

It is difficult to find the origin of intrauterine devices. Arabs are believed to have inserted stones into the uteruses of their camels to stop them becoming pregnant while on long journeys across the desert. The first IUD designed to prevent conception was a ring made from silkworm gut by Dr Richter in 1909. In the 1920s Ernst Graefenberg developed a silver ring known as the Graefenberg ring. In many countries contraception was illegal during this time, and antibiotics had not been developed to treat pelvic infection. Later, in 1934, Ota in Japan developed the Ota ring, a modification of the Graefenberg ring. In 1962 Dr Lippes introduced an IUD made of plastic called the Lippes Loop. It was not until 1965 that IUDs became available to women through Family Planning Clinics, and in 1969 copper wire was added to the IUD which was found to increase the efficacy of the device. The IUD is often referred to as the 'coil'.

Recently, newer IUDs have been introduced which have fewer side effects, increased efficacy and last up to 10 years. With the commencement of chlamydia screening IUDs have been given a new lease of life. The development of the intrauterine system Mirena, a progestogen-releasing intrauterine device, has meant that the choice of contraception has now widened.

THE INTRAUTERINE DEVICE

Explanation of method

An intrauterine device is inserted through the cervical canal and sits in the uterus. It has threads which hang down into the vagina, which a woman can check to make sure that the device is correctly positioned. It prevents pregnancy by impairing the viability of the sperm and ovum through the alteration of the fallopian tube and uterine fluids, and there is a foreign body reaction with an increase in leucocytes. This reduces the chances of the ovum and sperm meeting and impedes fertilization. The copper in IUDs is believed to be toxic to sperm and ovum.

Efficacy

The IUD is between 98 to nearly 100 per cent effective in preventing pregnancy, depending on the device. Newer IUDs like the T Safe 380A have a significantly lower failure rate at all stages of use with no pregnancies beyond eight years of use. The cumulative pregnancy rate at 12 years was 2.2 per 100 users, of which 0.4 were ectopic pregnancies (Dennis and Hampton, 2002). The GyneFix has a cumulative pregnancy rate of 0.5 at three years.

Disadvantages

- Menorrhagia.
- Dysmenorrhoea.
- Slightly increased risk of ectopic pregnancy if there is an IUD failure.
- Increased risk of pelvic infection (see p. 147).
- Expulsion of the IUD.
- Perforation of the uterus, bowel and bladder.
- Malposition of the IUD.
- Pregnancy caused by expulsion, perforation or malposition.

Advantages

- Effective immediately.
- No drug interactions.
- Reversible and highly effective.
- Not related to sexual intercourse.

UKMEC 4 unacceptable health risk: absolute contra-indication

- Pregnancy.
- Puerperal sepsis.
- Post-septic abortion.
- Gestational Trophoblastic disease with persistent elevated Beta HCG levels or malignant disease.
- Awaiting treatment for cervical cancer, endometrial cancer.
- Undiagnosed genital tract bleeding; once the cause has been diagnosed and treated an IUD may be inserted.
- Pelvic or vaginal infection; once treated an IUD may be fitted.
- Known pelvic tuberculosis.
- Allergy to components of IUD (e.g. copper).
- Wilson's disease.

- Less than four weeks post-partum.
- Ovarian cancer if inserting the device.
- Abnormalities of the uterus (e.g. bicornuate uterus, fibroids).
- Thrombocyopenia if inserting the device.
- Dysmenorrhoea and/or menorrhagia.
- HIV is classified as UKMEC3 for insertion and UKMEC2 for continuation unless the woman is using antiretrovirals and clinically well, whereupon both are UKMEC2. This is because of a reduced immune system caused by the HIV virus and, as a result, an increased risk of infection.

Range of method

There are 15 intrauterine devices available in the UK. Three different IUDs are shown in Fig. 11.1, and Table 11.1 lists all 15 together with details of their life span and construction.

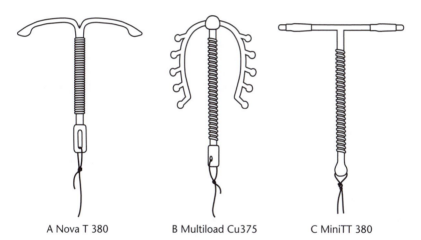

A Nova T 380   B Multiload Cu375   C MiniTT 380

Figure 11.1 Three different intrauterine devices

Side effects

- Menorrhagia.
- Dysmenorrhoea.

Table 11.1 Names and details of life span and construction of intrauterine devices

Device	Life span	Construction
Cu Safe T 300	5 years	300mm^2 copper wound around T-shaped stem
Multiload Cu375	5 years	Vertical stem 3.5cm in length; 375mm^2 of copper wound around
Multi-Safe 375	5 years	375mm^2 of copper wound around stem
Multi-Safe 375 short stem	5 years	375mm^2 of copper wound around stem
Flexi-T 300	5 years	300mm^2 of copper wound around stem
Flexi-T 380	5 years	380mm^2 of copper wound around stem
Nova T 380	5 years	380mm^2 of copper wire with silver core wound around stem
Load 375	5 years	U-shaped with 375mm^2 copper wire wound stem
Mini TT 380	5 years	380mm^2 wound around stem and copper collar around each distal portion of each arm
Neo-safe T 380	5 years	T-shaped with 380mm^2 copper wire wound stem
T Safe 380A Quickload	10 years	380mm^2 wound around stem and copper collar around each distal portion of each arm
TT 380 Slimline	10 years	380mm^2 wound around stem and copper collar around each distal portion of each arm
UT 380 Short	5 years	380mm^2 of copper wound around stem
UT 380 Standard	5 years	380mm^2 of copper wound around stem
GyneFix	5 years	Frameless IUD with 6 copper tubes each 5mm in length and 2.2mm in diameter with total 330 mm^2 of copper wound around stem and arms

Decision of choice

The decision of which IUD to insert will depend on the woman and the size of her uterus. The Flexi-T 380 is suitable for a uterine length of over 6cm, a Load 375 suitable for a uterine length of over 7cm while the Multiload Cu375 and the Multi-safe 375 are suitable for a uterine length of 6 to 9cm; and Mini TT 380 Slimline for a uterine length of 5cm. The Flexi-T 300 and Cu Safe T 300 are suitable for a woman with a uterine length of 5cm and over. The Nova T 380, T-safe 380A Quickload and TT 380 Slimline are suitable for a uterine length of between 6.5 and 9cm.

Research (Sivin and Stern, 1994) has shown that IUDs similar to the Ortho Gyne T 380 Slimline, which were compared to the Levonorgestrel IUD, have low pregnancy rates and low and declining rates of side effects, including pelvic infection. Research undertaken in Africa has confirmed that the pregnancy rates with copper T 380s are low (Farr and Amatya, 1994; Farr et al., 1996). Complications are most likely to occur at the insertion of an IUD. Perforation of the uterus, vasovagal shock, expulsion of the IUD, pelvic infection, pain and bleeding may occur following insertion or in the first year of use. The T-Safe 380A Quickload and TT 380 Slimline are the current favoured 380 IUDs available in the UK for insertions offering the highest efficacy and licensed for 10 years, which means that the risks associated with insertion are decreased, as the device does not require frequent changing. High-copper devices are believed to have increased contraceptive efficacy and the Nova T 380 has been found to have a cumulative pregnancy rate of 1.6. In further research the Nova T 380 was found to have a pregnancy rate of 2.0 and expulsion rate of 13.0 in five-year cumulative life-table event rates per 100 women (Cox, 2002).

The GyneFix is a frameless implant with no arms (Wildemeersch et al., 1994) which is fitted with an anchoring system to fix the anti-fertility components of the device permanently to the fundus of the uterus. It has been developed to reduce the risk of expulsion, and to lessen symptoms such as pain and bleeding, which are reasons for early removal. GyneFix has an expulsion rate of 0.6 per 100 GyneFix users at three years. However, there have been studies in the UK which have shown a higher expulsion rate. Masters et al. (2002) reported an expulsion rate at 12 months of 8.4 per cent (CI 5.8 – 13.4 per cent), and a study in Liverpool (Dennis et al., 2001) reported similar results. Masters and colleagues suggest that the difference in expulsion rates may be because original studies involved fitting the device in lithotomy position with ultrasound being performed immediately after insertion and further information on the importance of positioning should be investigated.

If a woman wishes to have an IUD fitted then the most suitable IUD will be one which has a long licence and high efficacy, resulting in lower risk of pelvic infection, expulsion and perforation. However, the IUD inserted will also depend on the size and shape of a woman's uterus, and the inserter will take into consideration all these factors when choosing which device to fit.

IUD counselling

When counselling a woman about an intrauterine device you should take a full past and present medical history, which will help to exclude any absolute contra-indications. Your discussion of the efficacy and risks of an IUD should include the following points.

1 Clients should be aware that their periods may be heavier and more painful. Menstrual periods may improve within a few months after insertion. If they are already painful and heavy another form of contraception may be more suitable, such as the Levonorgestrel IUS.

2 The risk of pelvic infection is slightly increased at insertion and for the first 20 days following it. Research has shown (Farley et al., 1992) that the risk of pelvic inflammatory disease (PID) was six times higher during the first 20 days following insertion, which emphasizes the need for screening and follow-up, and suggests that limiting changing IUDs will reduce the risk of infection. This research showed that there was a small or no risk of PID associated with long-term use of IUD, and that exposure to sexually transmitted diseases is the major cause of pelvic inflammatory disease rather than the type of IUD. An IUD will not protect any woman against sexually transmitted diseases and HIV, so these issues need to be approached with her. If your client is not in a permanent relationship and wishes to have an IUD inserted then her risk of exposure to sexually transmitted diseases may be higher and this should be discussed along with safer sex. Further reviews of the risks of infection with IUDs corroborate research by Farley et al. in 1992 (Drug and Therapeutics Bulletin, 2002).

This research indicates the necessity for routine screening. Current guidelines recommend screening for sexually transmitted infections prior to fitting (FSRH, 2007, 2009b). Routine screening for chlamydia and gonorrhoea should be ideally undertaken at a consultation prior to insertion for all women, so that the results are available at insertion. If a woman is having a post-coital IUD inserted, then prophylactic antibiotics should be given and screening for chlamydia and gonorrhoea should be performed at insertion. However, any woman who is experiencing symptoms of a sexually transmitted disease (e.g. dyspareunia (painful sexual intercourse), offensive discharge or on vaginal examination is found to have cervical excitation, pelvic pain or cervicitis) should undergo full screening for sexually transmitted diseases. If this is unavailable she should be referred to a genito-urinary medicine clinic.

You should encourage your client to attend early following an IUD insertion if she experiences any signs of vaginal infection such as abdominal pain along with pyrexia, so that full infection screening may be performed and antibiotics given early to prevent pelvic infection.

3　You should discuss with your client the risk of expulsion of the IUD which occurs in approximately one in 20 women (FSRH, 2007). This is most likely to occur following insertion, which is why it is important for your client to attend a follow-up consultation four to six weeks after insertion. It is also important to teach her to check her IUD threads every month after her menstrual period. If she can locate the end of the IUD device (which will feel like the end of a matchstick), she should be advised to use alternative contraception and return to see you.

4　There is a rare risk that during insertion the IUD may perforate the uterus or cervix; the risk of this happening is up to 2 per 1000 insertions (FSRH, 2007). If your client experiences low abdominal pain which continues following insertion with no improvement she should be advised to see a doctor.

5　Efficacy should be discussed with women, as no form of contraception is 100 per cent effective against pregnancy. If an IUD fails then there is a risk that a pregnancy may be an ectopic pregnancy, so you should advise women to return early so that this possibility can be excluded. If she experiences low abdominal pain which is persistent and either missed or scanty periods she should seek help immediately.

An IUD is usually inserted at the end of a menstrual period as the cervix is slightly opened at this time, making insertion easier. An IUD may be inserted up to five days after the earliest calculated day of ovulation as post-coital contraception. Following delivery of a baby a woman can have an IUD fitted six weeks postnatally. After a miscarriage or a termination of pregnancy an IUD may be inserted immediately if the pregnancy was less than 12 weeks.

It is a good idea to encourage women to eat prior to an IUD insertion, as they will then be less likely to feel faint following insertion. Many women allow themselves little or no time to recover from insertion. Following insertion they may experience cramp-like period pains and it may be helpful to warn them to allow more time for themselves and perhaps organize for someone else to pick up their children or leave work earlier that day.

The areas to be covered at counselling are summarized in Box 11.1.

BOX 11.1

Areas to be covered at counselling

- Full medical history.
- Check blood pressure, weight and height.
- Ensure client has contraceptive cover up until insertion.
- Take details of last menstrual period; exclude pregnancy if relevant.
- Discuss how an IUD works and its efficacy.
- Discuss insertion and removal procedure.
- Discuss side effects (e.g. heavy, painful periods).
- Discuss risks of insertion: expulsion, perforation, pregnancy and ectopic pregnancy.
- Perform bimanual examination to exclude contra-indications and take chlamydia and gonorrhoea swab.
- Discuss risk of infection and safer sex.
- Give literature on IUD.
- Organize date for insertion.

Insertion procedure

Prior to insertion the chlamydia and gonorrhoea result should be checked, information about the last menstrual period obtained to exclude an already present pregnancy, and a pregnancy test performed if required. Research (Guillebaud and Bounds, 1983) has shown that if 500mg of mefenamic acid is given orally prior to insertion there is a reduction in pain following insertion of an IUD. Women should empty their bladder prior to insertion, as this will make it easier for the inserter to feel the uterus abdominally and it will be more comfortable for the woman. Prophylactic antibiotics are no longer required for insertion or removal of intrauterine contraception in women who are at risk of bacterial endocarditis (FSRH, 2008a).

During the IUD insertion procedure your client may like to have someone to hold her hand and comfort her – this may be you, or a friend or partner. Prior to insertion a bimanual examination will be performed by the inserter to ascertain the size, position and direction of the uterus, and to check that there is no tenderness.

The skill and expertise of the inserter will help reduce any problems and side effects. However, if a woman would like to have local anaesthetic to reduce pain or has had problems with an IUD in the past, then this can be given with lignocaine gel or a paracervical block using lignocaine. She may need to be referred to a hospital clinic which specializes in difficult insertions and removals. If lignocaine is given via a paracervical block then the lignocaine ampoule should be warmed to 37°C, as this has been found to reduce the pain of the initial injection (Davidson, 1992).

Insertion of an IUD is performed by a 'non-touch technique', so a clean pair of gloves should be used following bimanual examination. A sterile speculum is inserted into the vagina and the cervix is located; this is cleaned with sterile cotton wool and antiseptic solution. A uterine sound is inserted into the uterus via the cervical canal to measure the length, direction and patency of the uterus. This may cause cramp-like period pains which should diminish when the uterine sound is removed. The cervix may be stabilized by Allis forceps or a tenaculum so that the IUD may be inserted more easily; these may cause some discomfort as the cervix is very sensitive. Next, the IUD is inserted through the cervical canal into the uterus. The threads of the IUD are shortened once it is in position and are tucked up behind the cervix. If there are any problems with an insertion your client should be referred to a specialist in IUDs.

Following insertion you should encourage your client to lie down and rest. Analgesia may be required for period pains. Sanitary towels should be used initially to reduce the risk of infection and because tampons may catch on the IUD threads which have not yet softened. Tampons may be used with the next menstrual period. Your client may experience bleeding initially. This is a good time to remind her of any initial problems and when to return; for example, if she experiences a change in her normal vaginal discharge or persistent abdominal pain.

You should teach your client how to check her IUD threads and encourage her to perform this check after each menstrual period. It is helpful to show your client a picture of the type of IUD she has had fitted, and how long it should remain *in situ*. Up-to-date written information should be given along with relevant telephone numbers of where to get help if needed. The IUD is effective immediately, so no additional contraception is required. An IUD procedure generally takes 10 minutes.

You will need to see your client in four to six weeks for an initial follow-up after insertion.

Vasovagal and anaphylaxis attacks

Vasovagal and anaphylaxis attacks are usually rare; however, it is important to have emergency equipment and clear guidelines available for such events. Your client may feel sweaty and complain of feeling faint or sick. She may look pale and her pulse may be slower. If the IUD insertion procedure is still in progress then this should be stopped, and the woman should be laid in a supine position with her head lowered and feet raised. If bradycardia persists then slow intravenous atropine 0.3 to 0.6mg/ml may be required. If the woman has difficulty breathing and there is loss of consciousness and absence of a carotid pulse, her airway should be maintained by using a pocket mask, and emergency services phoned and help summoned. She should be laid in the left lateral position, and if there is no central pulse then 0.5mg adrenaline 0.5ml of 1/1000 ml may be given by deep intramuscular injection. If there is no improvement this may be repeated at 10-minute intervals to the maximum of three doses. If required, cardiopulmonary resuscitation should be commenced. The woman should never be left unattended at any time (FSRH, 2010b).

Post-fitting

After fitting an IUD it is important to encourage women to return earlier than the scheduled four- to six-week appointment if they suffer any signs of infection, as the first 20 days after fitting are the highest infection time. If a client suffers from low abdominal pain or pyrexia then they should return early. It is good practice to encourage women to abstain from sexual intercourse for 48 hours so that the cervical mucus has returned to normal, helping to give some protection against transcending infection.

Subsequent visits

You should see your client four to six weeks post-IUD insertion to examine and discuss any problems she may have. Details of the last menstrual period should be taken, along with any problems she has experienced. You should ask about any pain or difficulties having sexual intercourse; can her partner feel the IUD threads? Has she been able to check her threads herself? This information will help you when you examine your client, as it will give you signs for infection and you will be able to re-teach your client how to check her threads if she is unable to do so. Your client should be examined with a speculum first so that the IUD threads may be observed. If the IUD threads appear too long they may be shortened. If a cervical smear is required this may be taken at this time. After the speculum examination a bimanual examination should be performed. If the tip of the IUD can be felt in the cervical os, which may not have been seen on speculum examination, then the IUD is too low in the uterine cavity and will need to be removed and a new device fitted. The cervix should be checked for cervical excitation by moving it gently from side to side. If pain is experienced while this is performed it may indicate infection or an ectopic pregnancy. If any signs of vaginal or pelvic infection are observed then you should refer your client to a genito-urinary medicine clinic for full infection screening if unavailable on site.

If there are no problems, the IUD should be checked every six months, but you should advise your client to return earlier if she experiences any problems.

Research (Bontis *et al.*, 1994) into copper IUDs and their pregnancy rates concluded that the pregnancy rate seemed to reduce if women were taught to self-check their IUD's threads and attended frequent follow-up appointments.

Removal procedure

An IUD may be removed at any time if a client does not mind becoming pregnant. However, if she wishes to avoid becoming pregnant alternative contraception should be commenced at least seven days prior to removal. If an IUD is being changed and a problem arises which prevents the insertion of a new device, then emergency hormonal contraception may be indicated for sexual intercourse prior to removal of the old device.

An IUD is removed by inserting a speculum into the vagina and locating the cervix, from which the IUD threads should be visible. Spencer Wells forceps are applied to the IUD threads and gentle traction is applied. The IUD should slowly descend into the vagina. If this does not happen this may be because the IUD has become embedded in the uterus, and you should refer your client to a specialist doctor experienced in difficult removals.

It is usually advised that IUDs are removed one year after the menopause, because there is concern that an IUD may cause pyometra (pus in the uterus) (CSAC, 1993b).

SELF-ASSESSMENT QUESTIONS

Answers and discussion at the end of the chapter.

1   Your client, who has an IUD *in situ*, is concerned that her menstrual period is two weeks late. What would you do?

2   A 45-year-old woman attends for her IUD to be changed. It was inserted five years previously and is a Nova T 380. What would you do in this situation, and what further information do you need to know?

3   A 35-year-old woman consults complaining of dyspareunia for two months. She is in a permanent relationship and has had an IUD *in situ* for two years with no previous problems. What would you do in this situation?

PROBLEMS ENCOUNTERED

If you or your client are unable to feel the IUD threads this may indicate that the IUD has been expelled or that the IUD has moved within the uterus, or perforated the uterus, taking the threads with it. You should advise your client to use alternative contraception as she may be at risk of pregnancy. However, she may already be pregnant and a pregnancy test should be performed to exclude this possibility, along with details of her last menstrual period and any signs of pregnancy which may be experienced. Extrauterine pregnancy should be excluded first by ultrasound scan. If your client has an intrauterine pregnancy and wishes to continue with the pregnancy the IUD may be left *in situ* if it is too difficult to remove. She should be advised that there is an increased risk of spontaneous abortion, premature labour or stillbirth. The IUD should be located after the birth if there are no complications.

If your client is not pregnant, the threads may be found using either Spencer Wells forceps or a thread retriever like the Retrievette or the Emmett (Bounds *et al.*, 1992b). If the threads are still lost, an ultrasound should be performed to locate the position of the IUD. If the IUD is found to be correctly positioned in the uterus, no further action is required. However, if it cannot be seen, a straight abdominal X-ray should be performed to exclude perforation.

Perforation

If an IUD perforates the uterus it may also perforate the bowel or bladder, and an ultrasound and X-ray will need to be taken to locate the device and a laparoscopy performed to remove the device.

Perforation is rare and more common in post-partum lactating women who have IUDs fitted. It is important to encourage women to return if they have any pain or discomfort which persists following insertion.

Infection

If a woman complains of any change in her normal discharge such as vaginal itching, soreness, offensive and/or increased discharge or pain, this should be investigated fully. If screening for all genital infections is unavailable you should refer women to their local genito-urinary medicine clinic where screening for chlamydia and sexually transmitted diseases will be performed.

Clients may wish to reduce the risk of infection by using condoms. Women may choose to use an IUD as a method of contraception and a condom to protect them against infection.

Ectopic pregnancy

If a woman complains of low abdominal pain which may be associated with a light, scanty or missed period, an ectopic pregnancy should be excluded. A pregnancy test and bimanual examination will need to be performed to confirm diagnosis; if this is confirmed she will need to be referred to her local hospital for emergency treatment. If diagnosis is unconfirmed by examination and pregnancy test, an urgent ultrasound will be performed to further exclude any likelihood of an ectopic pregnancy.

Pregnancy

If a woman who is pregnant with an intrauterine pregnancy and has an IUD *in situ* wishes to continue with the pregnancy, the IUD should be removed if the pregnancy is less than 12 weeks' gestation, the threads are visible and removal offers no resistance. There is a risk of spontaneous abortion if the IUD is removed but this is greater if the IUD is left *in situ*. It is not always possible to remove the IUD. Removal should only be attempted by an experienced doctor following discussion with the client.

Pain or bleeding

If a woman complains of pain or bleeding with an IUD this should be investigated fully first to exclude infection, perforation or ectopic pregnancy. Details about the bleeding pattern or pain should be ascertained, and a pregnancy test performed along with a bimanual examination and cervical smear test, screening for infection and ultrasound scan. If the pain continues and infection, perforation and ectopic pregnancy have been excluded, appropriate analgesia may be given, or changing an existing IUD to a different type may be a possible solution.

Actinomyces-like organisms (ALOs)

Actinomyces-like organisms are bacteria found in women with IUDs *in situ* by cytologists when cervical screening is performed. If a woman is symptomatic (e.g. she complains of pain, dyspareunia, or an increase in vaginal discharge), the IUD may be removed and sent for culture, with the IUD threads removed and a new IUD fitted. If the culture is negative to actinomyces a follow-up smear should be repeated. However, if the culture is positive to actinomyces, she will require antibiotic therapy which should be advised by the microbiology department.

If your client is asymptomatic, the presence of actinomyces-like organisms does not necessitate removal of the device; however, careful counselling, including symptoms which do necessitate removal and follow-up, should be discussed. After full counselling your client will be able to make an informed decision about whether she wishes to have the IUD removed or left *in situ*. This decision should be documented in her notes.

THE FUTURE

With research now indicating that IUDs may be left *in situ* longer, with less risk of infection and expulsion, it is likely that we will see licensing for IUDs being lengthened. Future IUDs are less likely to cause side effects of dysmenorrhoea and menorrhagia as designs of devices improve.

SEXUALITY AND ANXIETIES

Women who choose the IUD as their form of contraception do so often because it is 'out of sight and out of mind', meaning it requires little compliance or motivation from the woman and once *in situ* 'can be forgotten'. With an IUD there is no disruption to sexual intercourse, and therefore no loss of spontaneity. However, there are still many misconceptions held about IUDs by both men and women. Many people believe that the IUD causes infertility, infection and is an abortifacient. With such strong inaccurate views held it is not surprising that many women do not consider it as an initial form of contraception; this highlights the need for comprehensive counselling.

Many women are unaware of new IUDs with higher efficacy and longer life spans, which may take some women over difficult periods where other contraception is contra-indicated and the menopause is not too far off. Women may be concerned over the pain of insertion of an IUD. The use of pre-insertion analgesia and local anaesthetic can help to reduce this; however, the comfort and support of a nurse or a partner is vital.

A large proportion of women who have completed their families and do not wish to have any more children choose to have an IUD fitted; this may be because they see the risks of an IUD as relative now that their family is complete.

ANSWERS TO SELF-ASSESSMENT QUESTIONS

1   *Your client, who has an IUD* in situ, *is concerned that her menstrual period is two weeks late. What would you do?*

It is important to exclude pregnancy when your client has a delayed menstrual period. Details of the last episode of sexual intercourse and last menstrual period should be ascertained, and a pregnancy test performed if required. If your client is at risk of pregnancy and the test is negative, she will need to have a bimanual examination and ultrasound scan to exclude extrauterine or intrauterine pregnancy. If these are all negative your client may be reassured that she is not pregnant. If the test is positive she will need to have a bimanual examination and ultrasound scan to exclude extrauterine pregnancy. If the pregnancy is an ectopic pregnancy your client will need to be referred to the local hospital for emergency surgery. Once an extrauterine pregnancy has been excluded, how your client feels about the pregnancy will determine her care. If she does not want to proceed with the pregnancy and wishes to have a termination the IUD may be removed at the time of the termination procedure. If your client wishes to continue with the pregnancy and is under 12 weeks' gestation the IUD may be removed following discussion of the risks with her, if removal requires no resistance.

2   *A 45-year-old woman attends for her IUD to be changed. It was inserted five years previously and is a Nova T 380. What would you do in this situation, and what further information do you need to know?*

On discussion with the woman it may be decided to leave the IUD *in situ* for longer. She should be given as much information about keeping devices *in situ* past their licence so that she can make an informed decision.

It may be useful to find out when the woman's mother went through the menopause, as this may give an indication as to when she may do so. This will give a very rough idea of how long she will require contraception for. It is also important to find out how she feels about pregnancy and whether it will cause her more anxiety by not changing the IUD.

3   *A 35-year-old woman consults complaining of dyspareunia for two months. She is in a permanent relationship and has had an IUD* in situ *for two years with no previous problems. What would you do in this situation?*

It is important to find out more about the dyspareunia. Has there been a change in the women's discharge? Does she have pain at any other time? How long has she had dyspareunia? Can she describe the pain when she gets it?

She will need to be examined to exclude infection and to check the IUD. A bimanual and screening for all infections should be performed. If these are unavailable she will need to be referred. Until infection has been excluded she should be advised to use condoms to protect her partner against infection.

Once infection has been excluded and the IUD has been checked to be in the correct position, other causes of dyspareunia need to be investigated. There may be a psychosexual aspect to the dyspareunia which may need to be explored. Has the woman's relationship changed? Has she had dyspareunia before? Given time, this client may be able to talk about this difficult area.

THE INTRAUTERINE SYSTEM (IUS)

12

- Introduction and history
- The intrauterine system
- The future
- Sexuality and anxieties

INTRODUCTION AND HISTORY

In 1995 a new method of contraception, known as Mirena, was launched on the UK market. This product was developed by the Population Council and Leiras, a Finnish pharmaceutical company. Mirena is a Levonorgestrel-releasing intrauterine system (IUS). The development of the IUS has been a long process; the initial idea was considered in 1970. The process began with the development and production of a device which had a sleeve that released constant levels of the hormone Levonorgestrel over a long period of time. Mirena is also licensed for the treatment of primary menorrhagia which has relieved many women from horrendous menstrual problems when the only previous solution would have been a hysterectomy.

THE INTRAUTERINE SYSTEM

Explanation of the method

The intrauterine system (abbreviated to IUS) has a plastic T-shaped frame similar to a Nova T IUD but has a steroid reservoir around the vertical stem of the device containing the hormone Levonorgestrel. The device is 32mm in length and 4.8mm in diameter. It is inserted through the cervical canal into the uterus, where it sits releasing 20mcg of Levonorgestrel over 24 hours. Mirena is impregnated with barium sulphate which makes it radiopaque, and is licensed for five years (see Fig. 12.1).

The IUS prevents pregnancy through the suppression of the endometrium, making it unfavourable to implantation. In some women the IUS reduces ovarian function. It also causes the cervical mucus to thicken, making it impenetrable to sperm, and there is a foreign body reaction to the presence of the IUS.

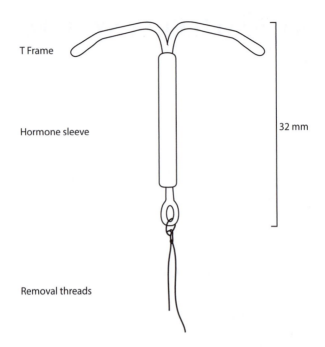

T Frame

Hormone sleeve

32 mm

Removal threads

Figure 12.1 Levonorgestrel IUS

Efficacy

The IUS has a mean failure rate of less than 0.2 per 100 woman years (Luukkainen, 1993). Published comparative multi-centre trials, which have covered more than 10,000 woman years (Luukkainen, 1993), have shown that the pregnancy rate has remained very low every year in the studies lasting more than five years.

Disadvantages

- Amenorrhoea.
- Irregular bleeding.
- Body of the IUS device is wider than other IUDs which means that dilatation of the cervix may be required.
- Expulsion of the IUS.
- Perforation of the uterus, bowel and bladder.
- Malposition of the IUS.
- Pregnancy caused by expulsion, perforation or malposition.
- Slightly increased risk of ectopic pregnancy if there is an IUS failure.
- Not suitable for post-coital use.

Advantages

- Reduction in menorrhagia.
- Reduction in dysmenorrhoea.
- Oligomenorrhoea and amenorrhoea.
- High efficacy.
- Reversible.
- Unrelated to sexual intercourse.

UKMEC 4 unacceptable health risk: absolute contra-indication

- Pregnancy.
- Undiagnosed genital tract bleeding; once the cause has been diagnosed and treated an IUS may be inserted.
- Pelvic or vaginal infection; once treated an IUS may be fitted.
- Puerperal sepsis.
- Septic abortion.
- Known pelvic tuberculosis.
- Suspected or confirmed endometrial or cervical malignancy.
- Current breast cancer.
- Gestational trophoblastic disease with persistent elevated Beta HCG levels or malignant disease.
- Serious side effects occurring on the COC which are not due to oestrogen.

UKMEC 3 risks outweigh the benefits of using method: relative contra-indication

- Current liver disease, liver adenoma or cancer.
- Current systemic disease.
- History of cerebrovascular accident, including TIA.
- Drugs which may interfere with the efficacy of the Mirena (e.g. enzyme-inducing drugs (FSRH, 2011b).
- Fewer than four weeks post-partum.
- Congenital or acquired uterine anomaly which distorts the fundal cavity, like fibroids.
- Breast cancer in the past five years.
- Ovarian cancer if inserting the IUS.
- HIV is classified as UKMEC 3 for insertion and UKMEC 2 for continuation unless the woman is using anti-retrovirals and is clinically well, whereupon both are UKMEC 2. This is because of a reduced immune system caused by the HIV virus and as result an increased risk of infection.

Range of method

Currently there is only one IUS available: Mirena.

Decision of choice

Women who are interested in having an IUS fitted should be carefully counselled about the side effects of the IUS. Functional ovarian cysts have been noted to be between 10 and 12 per cent with the IUS (Robinson *et al.*, 1989); most were asymptomatic and resolved spontaneously. The most common side effect with Mirena is irregular bleeding patterns, while other side effects were found initially in the first few months following insertion. Research (Andersson *et al.*, 1994; Sivin and Stern, 1994) has shown that the IUS significantly reduces bleeding and spotting, and is particularly useful for women requiring contraception and treatment for menorrhagia and dysmenorrhoea (Bounds *et al.*, 1993). Observational research has shown that Mirena has given significant symptomatic relief to women with adenomyosis (Ikomi and Pepra, 2002). Mirena is currently licensed for contraception, and treatment of Menorrhagia for five years, and prevention of endometrial hyperplasia during oestrogen replacement therapy licensed for four years.

When the IUS is removed, fertility returns to normal immediately and menstruation occurs within 30 days (Hollingworth and Guillebaud, 1994).

Side effects

- Some women may develop functional ovarian cysts.
- Breast tenderness.
- Acne.
- Headaches.
- Bloatedness.
- Mood changes.
- Nausea.
- Irregular bleeding.
- Amenorrhoea.

Drugs which affect the efficacy of the IUS

As the IUS release of progestogen is directly to the uterus and is unaffected by the metabolism of the liver, it is now believed that the risk of pregnancy is small. This is based on a small study (Bounds and Guillebaud, 2002) on women using Mirena taking anti-epileptic and other enzyme-inducing drugs, which came to no firm conclusions but suggested that any increased pregnancy risk – if it exists – fell within acceptable bounds.

IUS counselling

As with any method of contraception, the more information given to a client will not only ensure that she chooses the best method to suit her but also increases her future acceptability of the method. When counselling your clients about the IUS it is important to obtain a full medical history to exclude any contraindications. The side effects and efficacy of the IUS should be discussed, along with your client's contraceptive history. It is important that up until insertion a reliable form of contraception is used, as the IUS is not licensed as a post-coital form of contraception.

Many women will choose to have the IUS inserted because of its high efficacy and therapeutic effects on menorrhagia and dysmenorrhoea, even if it may make their already present acne or breast tenderness worse. This is often because they feel that their contraception and periods are the greatest of these problems, and that they will if necessary put up with other problems to alleviate these conditions. However, a woman who has very severe premenstrual problems and no problems with dysmenorrhoea or menorrhagia may find a new IUD more suitable, as this will not increase her premenstrual symptoms.

To increase the acceptability and continuation rates with the IUS it is important to discuss the hormonal side effects such as mastalgia, headaches, acne, hirsutism and mood swings. Clients may choose to accept these side effects because of the advantages of the IUS; however, they should also be reminded that the amount of Levonorgestrel through the IUS is only a fraction of the daily dose received through oral contraceptives so the side effects should be smaller with the IUS than with oral methods.

The IUS may cause oligomenorrhoea or amenorrhoea. There is a total reduction in menstrual blood loss because of the reduction in the thickness and vascularity of the endometrium caused by the presence of the IUS. This means that women may experience shorter, lighter, irregular menstrual periods and spotting. Spotting decreases with use and has been found to be less than four days at six months of use (Leiras, 1995). Woman should be warned that they may experience amenorrhoea which may cause some women anxiety; others, however, may see this as an advantage.

The risks of the IUS insertion procedure should be discussed along with the choice of having a local anaesthetic. It is important to talk about the possible need to dilate the cervix to introduce the IUS device, as this may be more painful than having an IUD device inserted, and occasionally the cervix will not dilate enough to allow insertion of the IUS, resulting in failure to fit the device. With all IUD and IUS procedures there is a small risk of perforation of the uterus or cervix; however, with an experienced inserter this risk will be lessened. There is a risk of partial or complete expulsion of the IUS, which is why it is important for it to have fundal positioning to reduce this possibility. The IUS has a low contraceptive failure rate, but if there is a method failure the pregnancy may be ectopic (Leiras, 1995). However, ectopic pregnancies are rare with the IUS, occurring in only 0.02 per 100 woman years (Andersson et al., 1994; Sivin and Stern, 1994) compared with 1.2 to 1.6 per 100 woman years for women using no contraceptive method (Andersson et al., 1994).

It is important to counsel your client about the possible risks if she becomes pregnant with an intrauterine pregnancy with the IUS in situ. Because of the high efficacy of the device there is limited information available about the outcome of a pregnancy with the IUS. Because of the local exposure to Levonorgestrel of an intrauterine pregnancy teratogenicity and virilization cannot be excluded, and termination of the pregnancy should be discussed. If this is discussed at counselling, then women will have the opportunity to think about this issue, and if they hold strong views against abortion they may wish to choose another method.

Prior to insertion of the IUS a bimanual examination should be performed to exclude any abnormalities of the uterine cavity such as fibroids, which will necessitate an ultrasound scan to confirm diagnosis prior to insertion. If a fibroid is causing the uterine cavity to be distorted, the IUS will be contra-indicated. Screening for chlamydia and gonorrhoea should be performed at this examination. If there is any suspicion of a genito-urinary infection full screening should be performed; if this is unavailable, your client will need to be referred to a genito-urinary clinic. Prophylactic antibiotics are no longer required for insertion or removal of intrauterine contraception in women who are at risk of bacterial endocarditis (FSRH, 2008a).

Areas to be covered at counselling are summarized in Box 12.1.

IUS insertion procedure

Prior to insertion of the IUS the chlamydia and gonorrhoea result should be checked, information about the last menstrual period obtained to exclude an already present pregnancy, and a pregnancy test performed if required, as the IUS is not licensed as a post-coital contraceptive. Fitting of the IUS is similar to that of the IUD. Research (Guillebaud and Bounds, 1983) has shown that if 500mg mefenamic acid is given orally prior to insertion there is a reduction in pain following insertion of an IUD. The women should empty her bladder prior to insertion as this will make it easier for the inserter to feel the uterus abdominally and it will be more comfortable for the woman. Emergency equipment should be available at all IUS and IUD insertions (see p. 150).

During the IUS insertion procedure your client may like to have someone present to comfort her. Prior to insertion a bimanual examination will be performed by the inserter to ascertain the size, position and direction of the uterus, and to check that there is no tenderness.

Your client may like to have a local anaesthetic to reduce pain, as the cervix may need to be dilated to fit the IUS. Anaesthesia can be given with a paracervical block using lignocaine. If lignocaine is given via a paracervical block the lignocaine ampoule should be warmed to 37°C, as this has been found to reduce the pain of the initial injection (Davidson, 1992). As an IUS insertion may involve dilatation of the cervix to introduce the device, the procedure should be carried out by an inserter who has received further training in IUS insertion and paracervical anaesthesia.

BOX 12.1

Areas to be covered at counselling

- Full medical history.
- Check blood pressure, weight and height.
- Ensure client has contraceptive cover up until insertion.
- Take details of last menstrual period; exclude pregnancy if relevant.
- Discuss how an IUS works and its efficacy.
- Discuss insertion and removal procedure.
- Discuss side effects (e.g. amenorrhoea, irregular menstrual cycle).

- Discuss risks of insertion: expulsion, perforation, pregnancy and ectopic pregnancy.
- Perform bimanual examination to exclude contra-indications and take chlamydia and gonorrhoea swab.
- Discuss safer sex.
- Give literature on IUS.

Insertion of an IUS is performed by a 'non-touch technique', so a clean pair of gloves should be used following bimanual examination. A sterile speculum is inserted into the vagina and the cervix is located; this is then cleaned with sterile cotton wool and antiseptic solution. A uterine sound is inserted into the uterus via the cervical canal to measure the length, direction and patency of the uterus. This may cause cramp-like period pains which should diminish when the uterine sound is removed. The cervix may be stabilized by Allis forceps or a tenaculum so that the IUS may be inserted more easily; these may cause some discomfort as the cervix is very sensitive. As the introducer to the IUS is wider than other IUDs – it is 4.8mm in diameter compared with a Nova T which is 3.7mm in diameter – Hegar dilators may need to be used to dilate the cervix to Hegar 5 or 6 in diameter. This may be uncomfortable and local anaesthetic can help alleviate this discomfort. Next, the IUS is inserted through the cervical canal into the uterus. The threads of the IUS are shortened once it is in position and are tucked up behind the cervix. Fundal positioning of the IUS is extremely important to reduce the risk of expulsion and to ensure the endometrium has full exposure to the progestogen in the device and maximum efficacy is obtained.

Following insertion you should encourage your client to lie down and rest. Analgesia may be required for period pains. Sanitary towels should be used initially to reduce the risk of infection and because tampons may catch on the IUS threads which have not yet softened. Tampons may be used with the next menstrual period. Your client may experience bleeding initially; this is a good time to remind her of any initial problems and when to return; for example, if she experiences a change in her normal vaginal discharge or persistent abdominal pain.

You should teach your client how to check her IUS threads and encourage her to perform this after each menstrual period. It is helpful to show your client a picture of the IUS and give up-to-date written information along with relevant telephone numbers of where to get help if needed. It is recommended that the IUS is fitted within the first seven days of the onset of menstruation, when no additional contraception is required. An IUS procedure generally takes ten minutes. The batch number of the IUS device and expiry date should be recorded in the woman's notes. You will need to see your client in four to six weeks' time for an initial follow-up after insertion. Your client should be advised to return earlier if she experiences pain, unusual vaginal discharge or pyrexia.

The IUS can be inserted immediately following a first-trimester abortion, and should be inserted six weeks post-partum following delivery. The IUS is not recommended as a first choice of contraception for women who are breast-feeding.

IUS removal procedure

Removal of the IUS is the same as the removal of an IUD and clients should not have had sexual intercourse within the past seven days. As fertility returns immediately, contraception should be discussed prior to removal (e.g. a diaphragm should be taught and fitted prior to removal if required).

Subsequent visits

Following insertion of the IUS an examination should be performed four to six weeks later, when blood pressure and weight should be taken. Details about menstrual cycle and any problems experienced should be ascertained. If your client has had amenorrhoea since fitting, a pregnancy test should be performed to exclude pregnancy; however, if there are no symptoms and the device is *in situ* you can reassure your client. A speculum and bimanual examination should be performed to check that the device is correctly positioned. The IUS threads should be visible on speculum examination. If the end of the IUS device is located (it feels like the end of a matchstick), the device is partially expelled. This is a good opportunity to show your client how to check her threads for the IUS if she is unable to do so.

If there are no problems and the device is correctly positioned, you should see your client in six months' time to check the device. However, you should remind your client when to return early; for example, if she experiences any persistent abdominal pain, unusual discharge, pyrexia or symptoms of pregnancy, or if she is in any way concerned.

PROBLEMS ENCOUNTERED

Lost threads

If you or your client are unable to feel the IUS threads this may indicate that the IUS has been expelled or that it has moved within the uterus or perforated the uterus, taking the threads with it. You should advise your client to use alternative contraception, as she may be at risk of pregnancy. However, she may already be pregnant and a pregnancy test should be performed to exclude this possibility, along with details of her last menstrual period and any signs of pregnancy which may be experienced. Extrauterine pregnancy should be excluded first by an ultrasound scan. If your client has an intrauterine pregnancy careful counselling will need to be given.

If your client is not pregnant, the threads may be found using either Spencer Wells forceps or a thread retriever. If the threads are still lost, an ultrasound should be performed to locate the position of the IUS. If the IUS is found to be correctly positioned in the uterus, no further action is required. However, if it cannot be seen a straight abdominal X-ray should be performed to exclude perforation.

Perforation

If an IUS perforates the uterus it may also perforate the bowel or bladder, and an ultrasound and X-ray will need to be performed to locate the device and a laparoscopy performed to remove the device. It is important to encourage women to return if they have any pain or discomfort which persists following insertion.

Ectopic pregnancy

If a woman complains of low abdominal pain which may be associated with a light, scanty or missed period, the possibility of an ectopic pregnancy should be excluded. A pregnancy test and bimanual examination will need to be performed to confirm diagnosis. If this is confirmed she will need to be referred to her local hospital for emergency treatment. If diagnosis is unconfirmed by examination and pregnancy test, an urgent ultrasound will be performed to further exclude any likelihood of an ectopic pregnancy.

Pregnancy

If a woman is pregnant with an intrauterine pregnancy and has an IUS *in situ*, careful counselling will need to be given about the possible risk of teratogenicity and virilization in the foetus, due to local exposure to Levonorgestrel. Due to lack of clinical experience with pregnancies with an IUS *in situ*, information is limited, and a termination of pregnancy should be discussed with your client.

Pain

If a woman complains of pain or bleeding with an IUS this should be investigated fully to exclude infection, perforation or ectopic pregnancy. Details about the bleeding pattern and pain should be ascertained, and a pregnancy test performed along with a bimanual examination and cervical smear test, screening for infection and an ultrasound scan.

Actinomyces-like organisms

Actinomyces-like organisms are a bacteria found in women with IUSs *in situ* by cytologists when cervical screening is performed. If a woman is symptomatic (e.g. she complains of pain, dyspareunia or an increase in vaginal discharge), the IUS may be removed and sent for culture, an STI screen completed and a new IUS fitted. If the culture is negative to actinomyces a follow-up smear should be repeated. However, if the culture is positive to actinomyces, she will require antibiotic therapy which should be advised by the microbiology department.

However, if your client is asymptomatic the presence of actinomyces-like organisms does not necessitate removal of the device. However, careful counselling, including advice about symptoms which do necessitate removal and follow-up, should be discussed. After full counselling your client will be able to make an informed decision about whether she wishes to have the IUS removed or left *in situ*. This decision should be documented in her notes.

Heavier or increased menstrual bleeding

Heavier or increased menstrual bleeding may indicate a partial expulsion of the IUS as the endometrium may not be having full exposure to Levonorgestrel; there will also be a decrease in efficacy of the device. You should advise your client to use alternative contraception (e.g. condoms). She should have a bimanual and speculum examination and a pregnancy test to exclude partial or complete expulsion and pregnancy. If this is not excluded, an ultrasound should be performed to locate the device.

SELF-ASSESSMENT QUESTIONS

Answers and discussion at the end of the chapter.

1   A 24-year-old woman consults requesting contraception after being refused a sterilization because of her age. She has three children and has had two miscarriages. None of her pregnancies have been planned and she finds it difficult to remember to take pills. What forms of contraception would be suitable for her?
2   What are the advantages of the IUS to a woman?
3   Who would be most suitable for IUS, and who do you think would be less suitable for an IUS and why?

THE FUTURE

The IUS has widened the field of contraception: not only does it offer excellent reversible contraception, but it has been shown to have qualities that make it extremely effective in the treatment of menorrhagia.

SEXUALITY AND ANXIETIES

With the introduction of the IUS the field of contraception has widened considerably. Not only is Mirena an extremely effective form of contraception but it offers many women treatment for dysmenorrhoea and menorrhagia; for many of these women the only relief from these symptoms would have been to have a hysterectomy. Mirena also offers women a suitable reversible option to sterilization, and has given women who are unable to use combined oral contraception another acceptable choice.

Many women who consult requesting Mirena have complex gynaecological and sexual histories – they perceive the IUS as being the answer to all their problems, which it may well be. Often these women have tried all other methods of contraception in an effort to solve their problem, with no success. However, some of these problems may be of a psychosexual nature, which the IUS will not alleviate. Given time, these anxieties may surface; if, however, they are not expressed, they may manifest as feelings of dissatisfaction with the method.

ANSWERS TO SELF-ASSESSMENT QUESTIONS

1   *A 24-year-old woman consults requesting contraception after being refused a sterilization because of her age. She has three children and has had two miscarriages. None of her pregnancies have been planned and she finds it difficult to remember to take pills. What forms of contraception would be suitable for her?*

From this history the client is looking for a method of contraception which has a high efficacy and which does not require compliance, as she finds it difficult to remember to take oral contraception. There are several methods available to her which fit this description: Depoprovera, IUDs and the IUS. Careful counselling should be given about each method and a detailed medical history taken, so that an informed decision may be made by the client. Some women may choose not to have Depoprovera owing to the requirement of having injections every 11 to 12 weeks. An IUD which has an eight-year licence may be a good choice, as might an IUS; both offer high efficacy and require little client compliance.

2   *What are the advantages of the IUS to a woman?*

The main advantages of the IUS to a woman are that her periods will become less painful and lighter; she may also experience no periods. If a woman has experienced anaemia from heavy periods this will also be alleviated. The IUS offers highly effective contraception with very low pregnancy rates, with the added benefit of being completely reversible. Finally, the IUS requires little compliance from a woman and is unrelated to sexual intercourse.

3   *Who would be most suitable for an IUS, and who do you think would be less suitable for an IUS and why?*

Those most suitable for the IUS are women:

- Requesting a method of contraception for a five-year period or longer.
- Who want a method with a high efficacy; they may have had a contraceptive failure or do not wish to become pregnant.

- Who may suffer from heavy or painful periods.
- Who may be unable to use other methods of contraception because of contra-indications (e.g. they have focal migraines and are unable to have the COC, or they may be unable to have the IUD due to heavy periods).

Women who are less suitable for the IUS include those who have experienced side effects with progestogen methods. These women may find the menstrual disturbances unacceptable. Some women find it disturbing to have amenorrhoea, as this is usually an indicator of pregnancy. Women are unable to have the IUS fitted if they are pregnant, have undiagnosed genital tract bleeding, or have a suspected malignancy or liver disorder. Women who have an abnormality of the uterus which distorts the uterus may be unable to have the IUS because the device may be expelled more easily. Women with circulatory disorders, thromboembolic disease, heart valve replacement and history of bacterial endocarditis should not have an IUS because they are absolute contra-indications. Other contra-indications are women who have had recent trophoblastic disease, chronic systemic disease or who are taking drugs which may interfere with the efficacy of the IUS.

EMERGENCY CONTRACEPTION

13

- Introduction and history
- Hormonal contraception
- Future contraception
- Intrauterine contraceptive devices
- The future
- Sexuality and anxieties

INTRODUCTION AND HISTORY

The first emergency contraceptives used to prevent pregnancy were douches; understandably these were not very successful. In the 1960s the first hormonal post-coital preparations used contained oestrogen only. This was replaced in 1983 by Yupze regimen, which contained oestrogen and progestogen and had to be taken within 72 hours of unprotected sexual intercourse and was known as Schering PC4.

Today there are three types of emergency contraception, two hormonal and one non-hormonal. The two hormonal emergency contraceptives licensed in the UK are the Levonorgestrel method which is available in the form of Levonelle One or Levonelle 1500, and the Ulipristal acetate method which is provided in the form of EllaOne. Levonelle One is also available over the counter in chemists. An intrauterine device may be inserted as a post-coital method, but this is not generally as well known as emergency hormonal methods with the general public or professionals.

In 1999 the government's Social Exclusion Unit produced the strategy for *Teenage Pregnancy* (Department of Health, 1999). The Social Exclusion Unit recommended an action plan to reduce teenage pregnancy rates in the UK, which involved a national campaign to change behaviour, joined-up action on local and national levels, better prevention of the causes of teenage pregnancy and increased support. The government followed this up with the *National Strategy for Sexual Health and HIV*, which identified certain areas of concern. These highlighted the need to improve education about sex and relationships, and contraceptive and genito-urinary medicine services (Department of Health, 2002). The reduction of misconceptions can only be achieved by increased education about contraception and sexual intercourse, as well as about when emergency contraception can be taken and where it is available.

Prior to giving emergency contraception, it is important to take a full medical history, including medications and allergies. In order to ascertain what methods the client is eligible for, you will need to have detailed information about the date of the last menstrual period, and when the client has had unprotected sexual intercourse and earlier emergency contraception administered during the current cycle.

Emergency contraception has two main methods: hormonal contraception and intrauterine contraception.

HORMONAL CONTRACEPTION

Levonorgestrel method

Explanation of the method

The Levonorgestrel method prevents pregnancy in a number of ways and it is not completely understood how it does this. Depending where in the cycle it is administered it can inhibit ovulation by preventing follicular rupture or cause luteal dysfunction. If the Levonorgestrel method is given prior to the luteinizing surge it has been found to cause ovulatory dysfunction in the subsequent five to seven days. The Levonorgestrel method has been shown to be less effective the closer to ovulation it is given (FSRH, 2012a). There is no evidence of any pregnancy complications or congenital malformations associated with this method.

Efficacy

The efficacy of the Levonorgestrel method varies between 97 and 99 per cent in preventing pregnancy with the lower efficacy rate applying to mid-cycle unprotected sexual intercourse which has the greatest risk of pregnancy. Both hormonal methods have been found to be less effective if the unprotected sexual intercourse is just before ovulation, or there are further episodes of unprotected sexual intercourse (Prabakar and Webb, 2012).

However, not all episodes of unprotected sexual intercourse result in pregnancy. It is estimated from an analysis of published trials that this regimen's efficacy reduces the probability of pregnancy by 86 per cent (FFPRHC, 2003). Although this is a huge reduction in the risk of pregnancy, it is no replacement for effective ongoing contraception. An episode of unprotected sexual intercourse on any day in the menstrual cycle has an overall risk of pregnancy of 2 to 4 per cent (Trussell and Stewart, 1992; FFPRHC, 2003) and will be higher around ovulation at between 20 and 30 per cent (FFPRHC, 2003).

Disadvantages

- Does not provide future contraception.
- Next menstrual period may be early or delayed.
- Nausea and vomiting.

Advantages

- Effective in preventing pregnancy.
- Under the woman's control.

UKMEC 4 unacceptable health risk: absolute contra-indication

■ Pregnancy.
■ Although the UK Medical Eligibility Criteria advise that there are no medical contra-indications to the Levonorgestrel method, caution should applied to women with acute active porphyria, severe liver disease and allergy to Levonorgestrel (FSRH, 2009a).

Range of method

Levonelle 1500 has one tablet made of the hormone progestogen, containing 1500mg of Levonorgestrel. It is available in the form of Schering Levonelle One for post-coital use, with an instruction leaflet; it is also available over the counter from pharmacists for £24.

The Levonorgestrel method should be commenced within 72 hours of the earliest episode of unprotected sexual intercourse. Although this regimen is only licensed for 72 hours it may be given later (FFPRHC, 2003; FSRH, 2012a). Recent research has shown that the Levonorgestrel method is effective up to 96 hours; however, 96 hours to 120 hours is still unknown (FSRH, 2012a). Previous research into Levonelle One given 73 to 120 hours after unprotected sexual intercourse showed that 60 to 63 per cent of expected pregnancies were prevented; the responsibility for this unlicensed use will be the prescriber's. This should be discussed fully with the client, along with the alternative choice (an IUD) so that she is able to make an informed decision.

Side effects

■ Nausea.
■ Vomiting.
■ Fatigue.
■ Headaches.
■ Dizziness.
■ Breast tenderness.

How to take the Levonorgestrel method

The Levonorgestrel method is prescribed as Schering Levonelle One or Levonelle 1500. Schering Levonelle One and Levonelle 1500 contains one tablet. One tablet should be taken within 72 hours from the earliest episode of unprotected sexual intercourse. As emergency contraception can make women feel nauseated, it is a good idea to advise them to take the tablet with or after food.

If the client vomits within two hours after taking Schering Levonelle One, she will need to return for a repeat prescription and take the dose immediately within the 72 hours. If a woman suffers from severe vomiting, an IUD may need to be considered.

Drugs which affect the efficacy of the Levonorgestrel method regimen

There is limited evidence about the effect of enzyme-inducing drugs like Rifampicin on Levonorgestrel's efficacy, but it is currently recommended that two tablets of Levonelle 1500 (1.5mg of Levonorgestrel) be given, increasing the dose to one stat dose of 3mg of Levonelle 1500. This is outside the product licence so would need to be named-patient prescribed by a doctor. Levonelle 1500's effectiveness is not believed to be reduced by non-enzyme-inducing antibiotics, as progestogens do not undergo significant reabsorption in the bowel, so there is no need to increase the dosage of Levonelle 1500 if a woman is taking antibiotics (FSRH, 2011b). However, caution is advised when prescribing Levonelle 1500 to women on Warfarin treatment, as the effects of Warfarin may be decreased or increased with Levonelle 1500.

Ulipristal acetate method

Explanation of the method

Ulipristal acetate prevents pregnancy by inhibiting or delaying ovulation depending when in the cycle it is administered. It is believed that Ulipristal acetate can prevent ovulation after the Luteal surge has started and delay follicular rupture up to five days later. If Ulipristal acetate is administered after implantation has occurred there is limited evidence of the effects on pregnancy and teratogenicity.

Ulipristal acetate is a synthetic progesterone which binds to human progesterone receptors; as a result it blocks the action of progestogen and may reduce the efficacy of contraceptives containing progestogen. Ulipristal acetate has a high affinity for glucocorticoid receptor and antiglucocortoid effects have been observed in animals. It is therefore not recommended for use with women suffering from severe asthma insufficiently controlled by oral glucocorticoids (FSRH, 2012a).

Efficacy

Ulipristal acetate, if given within the first 72 hours after unprotected sexual intercourse, is as effective as the Levonorgestrel method (FSRH, 2012a). However, research has shown that Ulipristal acetate is more effective than the Levonorgestrel method between 72 and 120 hours. Glasier's research showed that in randomized efficacy studies which compared EllaOne and Levonelle 1500, of 844 women given EllaOne and 852 women given Levonelle 1500 there were 15 pregnancies (1.8%) with EllaOne and 22 pregnancies (2.6%) with Levonelle 1500 within 72 hours of unprotected sexual intercourse. Two hundred and three women were given emergency contraception beyond 72 to 120 hours; 97 women were given EllaOne and 106 Levonelle 1500, and three pregnancies occurred, all with Levonelle 1500 (Glasier et al., 2010).

Disadvantages

- Does not provide future contraception.
- Next menstrual period may be early or delayed.
- Nausea and vomiting.

Advantages

- Effective in preventing pregnancy.
- Under the woman's control.

UKMEC 4 unacceptable health risk: absolute contra-indication

- Pregnancy.
- Allergy to constituents.
- Severe asthma controlled by glucocorticoids.
- Renal and hepatic impairment.
- Repeated doses in the same cycle.
- Galactose intolerance and lapp lactose deficiency or glucose-galactose malabsorption.
- Breast-feeding.

Range of method

Ulipristal acetate method contains 30mg of Ulipristal acetate (UPA) and is given within 120 hours of unprotected sexual intercourse. It is licensed under the name EllaOne.

Side effects

- Nausea.
- Vomiting.
- Fatigue.
- Headaches.
- Menstrual disorders.

How to take the Ulipristal acetate method

The Ulipristal acetate method is prescribed as EllaOne and contains one tablet. The tablet should be taken within 120 hours of the earliest episode of unprotected sexual intercourse. As emergency contraception can make women feel nauseated, it is a good idea to advise them to take the tablet with or after food.

If the client vomits within three hours after taking EllaOne she will need to return for a repeat prescription and take the dose immediately within the 120 hours. If a woman suffers from severe vomiting an IUD may need to be considered.

Breast-feeding women are advised not to breast-feed and to discard expressed milk for five days after taking EllaOne, as Ulipristal is excreted in milk (FSRH, 2013).

Drugs which affect the efficacy of the Ulipristal acetate method

Liver enzyme-inducing drugs reduce the efficacy of progestogen. There is no current advice for EllaOne, but advice for Levonelle 1.5mg is to increase the dose by 100 per cent, so a stat dose orally of Levonelle 3mg two 1.5mg tablets should be given within 72 hours.

The current advice with liver enzyme-inducing drugs and Ulipristal acetate is that it should not be used while a woman is taking these drugs or within 28 days after they have been taken. The Clinical Effectiveness Unit does not recommend increasing the dose of Ulipristal acetate (FSRH, 2012a).

Women who are taking drugs which increase gastric pH such as antacids, histamine H2 antagonists and proton pump inhibitors may reduce the plasma concentration of Ulipristal acetate and as a result reduce the efficacy – EllaOne should not be prescribed in these cases.

Decision of choice

The hormonal method of post-coital contraception is a safe effective method. When deciding which method to choose, once a careful history has been taken and detailed counselling given, it is important to ascertain when unprotected sexual intercourse has taken place. If this is beyond 72 hours, the Levonorgestrel method will not be the most effective method of emergency contraception and the Ulipristal acetate method should be considered. If a woman has an absolute contra-indication to the hormonal method, an IUD should be considered. Women wishing to use the IUD as a method of contraception may have this fitted as an emergency method; however, it is important to remember that occasionally an IUD is unable to be fitted and this may be more likely to occur with nulliparous women. Another factor to remember when choosing which method to use is the risk of genito-urinary infection which may be the result of the unprotected sexual intercourse. Because of this factor, if the episode is within 72 hours, taking the hormonal method may be of less risk to the woman than fitting an IUD.

The Levonorgestrel method is licensed for up to 72 hours after unprotected sexual intercourse; evidence shows that Levonelle is effective up to 96 hours; however, the efficacy between 96 and 120 hours (five days) after unprotected sexual intercourse is unknown (FSRH, 2012a). Although randomized trials investigated the use of Levonorgestrel beyond 72 hours and found that 60 to 63 per cent of expected pregnancies were prevented, few women used this method after 72 hours, giving wide confidence intervals (Von Hertzen et al., 2002). Ideally, women should take the Levonorgestrel method within 72 hours; however, if a woman is beyond this time an IUD is the most effective form of post-coital method. If a woman is beyond 72 hours following unprotected sexual intercourse but within five days of its occurrence she may be suitable for the Ulipristal acetate method, and this together with a post-coital intrauterine device should be considered and discussed with her. The Levonorgestrel method may be given more than once in the cycle, whereas this is not recommended for the Ulipristal acetate method. There may be occasions when a client is unsuitable for a post-coital IUD; for example, if a women has PID, has been raped or feels unable to go through the procedure of an insertion, giving the Levonorgestrel method late may then be indicated.

Counselling

Women who attend for emergency contraception are often very anxious and embarrassed; they may show varying emotions from anger to guilt. Sexual intercourse may not have been with consent, and a woman may feel shocked and distressed. Often the situation in which women find themselves feels threatening to them, and their feelings of anger and guilt, etc. are aimed at you. You may come across women who have difficulty in answering some of the personal questions you need to ask. 'Why do you need to know that?' is not an uncommon response. It is important to allow enough time for this consultation and explain why you need to ask such personal questions. It is also a good idea to allow your client time to read through up-to-date literature about emergency contraception beforehand so that you can build on this knowledge and answer any questions it may initiate.

Often clients fail to tell you about earlier episodes of unprotected sexual intercourse, as they do not feel they are at risk of pregnancy from these episodes. Women often believe that unprotected sexual intercourse around the end of their menstrual period will be safe, so this can be a good opportunity to explain about ovulation and how it is possible for sperm to live in the body for up to seven days (Guillebaud, 1999). If your client has had earlier unprotected sexual intercourse the hormonal method will be contra-indicated, but it may be possible to fit an IUD if it is within five days of the calculated date of ovulation. It is useful when recording details about episodes of earlier unprotected sexual intercourse to chart these on a menstrual calendar along with details of when the first day of the last menstrual period occurred and length of normal menstrual cycle; this will also make calculating ovulation easier. Often while you are doing this it triggers clients' memories and they may remember further episodes of unprotected sexual intercourse.

If there is any doubt that your client's last menstrual period was not normal, a pregnancy test should be performed to exclude pregnancy. Some women (mistakenly) believe that emergency contraception will be effective in preventing an existing pregnancy.

When counselling men and women about emergency contraception it is important to discuss the efficacy and side effects of post-coital contraception. Sometimes women decide not to have emergency contraception after they have received counselling; this usually happens when the woman is in a stable relationship and willing to accept the risk of pregnancy, or if the risk is low. Occasionally it is not possible to give post-coital contraception because the woman has had multiple episodes of unprotected sexual intercourse which exceed 72 hours and are beyond five days of calculated ovulation so that an IUD cannot be inserted. This situation is often made worse if the woman has had unprotected sexual intercourse with someone other than her regular partner. As health professionals you want to make 'everything better'. This is a situation when you are unable to do this, and this can not only be very difficult for the client but also for the nurse. What you may find hardest is that you can give no guarantees – you cannot reassure the woman that she won't become pregnant, because there is a real risk that she may become pregnant. You also need to approach the issue of safer sex and contraception, which may at this time be an area she has not thought about. Listening to the woman's distress and anxieties are the main functions of the nurse. It is often hard not to falsely reassure a woman in this situation, but being there and listening to the pain your client is suffering are far more important to her. An appointment should be made after your client's estimated next menstrual period so that a pregnancy test can be performed; if possible this appointment should be with you.

Sometimes the request for emergency contraception has been precipitated by rape. Shock may prevent a woman from attending early for emergency contraception, which may mean that an IUD is indicated or that you are unable to give emergency contraception. It is vital that a woman has screening for all genito-urinary infections and HIV from a specialist clinic. Rape counselling should be offered. Women may feel that they do not want this at the time, but information and telephone numbers should be given in case they wish to follow this up in the future.

Many different women and men attend for emergency contraception. They may be women in their forties whose unprotected sexual intercourse may cause a change in their contraceptive practice to a permanent method like sterilization in the future; they may feel that they should have known better and be embarrassed. Other clients may be young men and women who may be under the age of 16 and have recently commenced sexual activity. They may be anxious that the information they give may not stay confidential, and are embarrassed and humiliated by the personal questions that are asked. Many younger clients feel that they will be judged by the health professionals they see. It has usually taken a great deal of courage for them to attend, and the impression they gain from this encounter will establish whether they attend in the future. Their confidentiality should be respected unless the health, safety or welfare of someone other than the client is at serious risk (BMA *et al.*, 1993). Occasionally young clients are being sexually abused and, if given time for a rapport to be established, they may return to confide in you.

A full medical history of the client and family should be completed to exclude any contra-indications. If a client has previously had emergency contraception it is useful to know if she has had any problems such as vomiting, etc. so that appropriate advice can be given. If a woman has used emergency contraception repeatedly because of a contraceptive failure or because no contraception has been used, then future contraception should be discussed carefully. If your client has had a contraceptive failure, teaching her how to avoid this will help reduce the necessity of emergency contraception in the future.

It is extremely important that women continue to use either a condom or abstain until their next period, as hormonal emergency contraception will not prevent a woman from becoming pregnant during the remaining part of the cycle. If a woman has a further episode of unprotected sexual intercourse then she may be more at risk of pregnancy, because the Levonorgestrel regimen can delay ovulation, resulting in this episode now being when she is ovulating! Women should be advised that if this situation occurs they need to return for further treatment. There is often a great deal of anxiety about giving repeated doses of hormonal emergency contraception but, as long as the latest episode is within 72 hours and there are no other contra-indications, the Levonorgestrel method may be prescribed.

ACTIVITY

Do you know where your clients can receive emergency contraception if you are unavailable? What about weekends and bank holidays?

Blood pressure, height and weight should be checked; a pelvic examination is not required with the hormonal method unless pregnancy is suspected or screening for infection. Anyone who has unprotected sexual intercourse puts themselves at risk of sexually transmitted disease and HIV, and if full infection screening is unavailable they should be referred to their local genito-urinary medicine clinic.

When giving emergency contraception to clients it is important to explore their attitudes towards pregnancy, and to discuss the possible failure of emergency contraception. There is no evidence to indicate that the Levonorgestrel method is not safe in pregnancy; however, at present there is limited evidence to show that the Ulipristal acetate method is safe in pregnancy. This method is therefore not recommended with multiple episodes of unprotected sexual intercourse, as it may carry a risk of teratogenicity (FSRH, 2012a); however, no one can guarantee a normal outcome in any pregnancy. You should advise your client that her next menstrual period may be early, on time or later than expected. If it is not a normal period or is absent she should return with a urine sample so that a pregnancy test may be performed. There is a risk in early pregnancy of an ectopic pregnancy. If a woman experiences abdominal pain she should be advised to seek medical attention. It is good practice to offer women the opportunity to return three to four weeks later; this gives you the opportunity to review any problems with contraception.

As clients are often very anxious when they consult, all the information you give should be backed up by up-to-date information, as clients are more likely to forget details if they are anxious. It is useful to have up-to-date information available about other local clinics which offer emergency contraception. If, for example, you give emergency contraception on a Friday and the client vomits and requires a second dose of pills, it is useful to give her addresses of alternative clinics if you are not available on the Saturday. It is a good idea to advertise this information in your waiting room and make it available to other staff in case they receive telephone enquiries.

The areas to be covered at counselling are summarized in Box 13.2.

FUTURE CONTRACEPTION

If a woman is happy to use condoms she needs to continue with these until she changes to another method. If, however, she has been given emergency contraception and wants to start another method, she can continue with condoms until her next period and start a hormonal method on the first day of her next period, and she will be safe straight away. Alternatively she could 'quick start' onto a hormonal method; this is an unlicensed practice which is endorsed by the Faculty of Sexual and Reproductive Healthcare. You need to involve your client in the discussion about this practice, and be reasonably certain that she is not already pregnant. Following Levonelle 1500 she could start the combined pill the next day and will need to use extra precautions for seven days (with Qlaira this will be for nine days). As her period will not be at its expected time, she should be advised to do a pregnancy test in three weeks' time. If the client wants to commence the progestogen-only pill she could also start this the following day after taking Levonelle 1500 and she should be advised to use extra precautions for two days and take a pregnancy test in three weeks' time.

EllaOne may reduce the efficacy of progestogen. Because of this, if you are quick starting a woman on contraception she should be advised to take EllaOne, and start the progestogen-only pill the following day, taking extra precautions for nine days and a pregnancy test in three weeks' time. If she wishes to commence the combined pill she should be advised to take EllaOne, and start the combined pill the next day and use extra precautions for 14 days (if it is Qlaira, 16 days) and a pregnancy test in three weeks' time. As quick starting is outside the product licence, this will need to discussed with the woman; however, it is endorsed by the Faculty of Sexual and Reproductive Healthcare Clinical Effectiveness Unit (FSRH, 2012a).

If a woman wishes to commence the injectable, the implant or the IUS, these should be started with the next period. Alternatively she could commence the progestogen-only pill Cerazette the next day after emergency contraception, using extra precautions either for two or nine days, depending on whether she takes Levonelle or EllaOne, and return in three weeks for a pregnancy test and commencement of the injectable, implant or IUS, if the test is negative.

BOX 13.1

Quick starting contraception following Levonelle 1500 and EllaOne

	Commence the combined pill the next day. Pregnancy test in 3/52.	Commence Qlaira the next day. Pregnancy test in 3/52.	Commence the progestogen-only pill the next day. Pregnancy test in 3/52.
Levonelle 1500 given stat	Extra precautions for 7/7.	Extra precautions for 9/7.	Extra precautions for 2/7.
EllaOne given stat	Extra precautions for 14/7.	Extra precautions for 16/7.	Extra precautions for 9/7.

Follow-up appointment

You should offer to see your client three to four weeks following post-coital contraception to check that she has had a normal menstrual period. If this is shorter or lighter than normal a pregnancy test should be performed to exclude pregnancy. This is an excellent opportunity to encourage sexually transmitted infection screening.

BOX 13.2

Areas to be covered at counselling

■ First day of last menstrual period and details of menstrual cycle length.
■ Was her last menstrual period normal – is there any possibility that she may already be pregnant? Do you need to perform a pregnancy test?
■ Time and date of earliest unprotected sexual intercourse – how many episodes of unprotected sexual intercourse have there been since the first day of the last period?
■ Has your client any contra-indications to emergency contraception?

- What contraception was used? Is your client happy to continue with this method or does she want to try another method?
- Has she had emergency contraception before? Did she have any problems with it (e.g. vomiting)?
- Record blood pressure.
- Does your client understand how to take the emergency contraception and know when she needs to return?
- Has your client read and been given up-to-date information about emergency contraception, and does she have contact numbers if she vomits or has a problem?

INTRAUTERINE CONTRACEPTIVE DEVICES

Explanation of the method

An IUD works as a post-coital method by preventing implantation and may also block fertilization. As pregnancy and implantation does not occur until five to seven days after fertilization, this means that the IUD does not act as an abortifacient.

Efficacy

The IUD is almost 100 per cent effective in preventing pregnancy post-coitally.

Disadvantages

- Slightly increased risk of ectopic pregnancy if there is an IUD failure.
- Increased risk of pelvic infection.
- Expulsion of the IUD.
- Perforation of the uterus, bowel and bladder.
- Malposition of the IUD.
- Pregnancy caused by expulsion, perforation or malposition.
- Minor surgical procedure.

Advantages

- Effective in preventing pregnancy.
- Unrelated to partner.
- IUD may be kept *in situ* and used as a form of contraception for the future.
- Longer time span of up to five days.

UKMEC 4 unacceptable health risk: absolute contra-indication

- Pregnancy.
- Present pelvic, vaginal infection, although an IUD may be inserted in special circumstances with antibiotic cover.
- Undiagnosed genital tract bleeding.
- In persistently elevated Beta-HCG levels or malignant disease an IUD should not be inserted.
- Less than four weeks post-partum an IUD should not be inserted.

Range of method

The type of IUD usually used post-coitally is a Nova T 380, but a Multiload or Flexi-T 300 or 380 or T-safe 380A or TT380 may be used.

Side effects

- Menorrhagia.
- Dysmenorrhoea.
- An IUD may be difficult to fit in nulliparous women.

Decision of choice

An IUD may be fitted as a form of emergency contraception up to five days after the calculated date of ovulation. It provides contraception for the rest of the month, and if a woman wishes can either be left *in situ* after her next menstrual period or removed. Women who have a contra-indication to the hormonal method may be able to have an IUD fitted, along with women who cannot accept the failure rate of the hormonal method.

Counselling

Women who have a post-coital IUD fitted may be more anxious than women having routine IUDs fitted, which can make insertion difficult. As they have had less time to prepare themselves for the procedure, it is important to allow them time to ask any questions and discuss the insertion procedure, risks, efficacy, and advantages and disadvantages of the IUD. You should complete a full medical history which will enable you to eliminate any contra-indications to the procedure and, with the aid of a menstrual calendar and information on the first day of the last menstrual period, estimate the calculated date of ovulation. If there is any possibility of your client being pregnant you should complete a pregnancy test, and a bimanual examination will need to be performed to exclude pregnancy.

If your client has not eaten recently it is preferable that she has something to eat prior to insertion; this will reduce the chances of her feeling faint. Analgesia may be given, and will be absorbed faster if a client has eaten. Although all this may seem time-consuming it will have the effect of reducing anxiety in the woman, which will aid insertion of the device and will reduce pain felt following insertion.

Prior to fitting an IUD, screening for chlamydia and gonorrhoea should be performed. As the result will not be available for the insertion of a post-coital IUD, prophylactic antibiotics are recommended. If there are signs of cervical or pelvic infection full screening for infection is recommended, especially in the case of rape, which may necessitate referral to a genito-urinary medicine (GUM) clinic. When referring your client to a GUM clinic, you may find it possible for the post-coital IUD to be inserted following screening at the clinic.

The IUD procedure is the same as for a routine IUD procedure. Your client should be shown how to check her IUD threads, and be advised that she may experience some bleeding and period-like pains after fitting. She should be encouraged to avoid tampons and use sanitary towels immediately after insertion in case these catch on the threads. If she experiences persistent pain she should be advised to seek medical attention to exclude an ectopic pregnancy. It is vital to give up-to-date literature and emergency telephone numbers to your client. A follow-up appointment should be made three to four weeks after insertion.

Follow-up appointment

You should see your client three to four weeks following insertion to check that she has had a normal menstrual period. If this is shorter or lighter than normal a pregnancy test should be performed to exclude pregnancy. If she is having her IUD removed with her period, alternative contraception should be commenced seven days prior to removal. Hormonal contraception is usually commenced on day 1 of a normal period. The COC should be commenced on day 1 of a normal menstrual period with no additional precautions required. The POP should be commenced on day 1 of a normal menstrual period, with no additional precautions required. Once alternative contraception has been established, the IUD may be removed. If, however, she would like to continue with the IUD as her method of contraception the IUD should be checked.

PROBLEMS ENCOUNTERED WITH EMERGENCY CONTRACEPTION

Vomiting with the hormonal contraception

It is a good idea to try to prevent vomiting prior to its incidence. Women should be encouraged to avoid taking the emergency contraception on an empty stomach. An anti-emetic like motilium (Domperidone) may be prescribed if vomiting occurs with a repeat dose of the emergency hormonal contraception. If vomiting is severe an IUD may need to be considered.

Previous use of the Levonorgestrel method in the cycle and a further episode of unprotected sexual intercourse

The Levonorgestrel regimen may be given if it has been previously used in the cycle but the Ulipristal acetate method should not be used more than once in a cycle. It is important to check that the previous dose was taken correctly and no other unprotected sexual intercourse has taken place other than the recent episode. If this is the case, an IUD may be indicated if it is within five days of the earliest calculated date of ovulation.

SELF-ASSESSMENT QUESTIONS

Answers and discussion at the end of the chapter.

1 A woman with a regular cycle of 4/25 days attends requesting emergency contraception. It is 100 hours since the first episode of unprotected sexual inter-course, and she is now on day 20 of her cycle. Can you give her emergency contraception?

2 What are the indications for emergency contraception?

THE FUTURE

Guidelines are regularly updated by the Clinical Effectiveness Unit on Emergency Contraception by The Faculty of Sexual and Reproductive Healthcare's recent guidance (FSRH, 2012a). It is important that all health professionals keep them-selves up to date with changes to these guidelines.

SEXUALITY AND ANXIETIES

Men and women consulting for emergency contraception are often extremely anxious. This is exacerbated by meeting someone, often in these circumstances for the first time, to discuss intimate details of their sex life, which can make it a harrowing situation. However, if handled appropriately it can be the beginning of a relationship that will give clients a richer knowledge and awareness of sexual health. In adopting an empathetic approach towards your clients that does not judge their sexual practices you will encourage them to consult in the future.

An episode of unprotected sexual intercourse (UPSI) often precipitates a change in contraceptive method, although clients often fail to mention this. When changing methods it is useful to ask about unprotected sexual intercourse, as this may affect when a new method may be commenced and may also mean that emergency contraception can be discussed.

Many women perceive the hormonal method to have more risks than regularly taking the combined pill (Ziebland *et al.*, 1996), and often accept the greater risks of an abortion by avoiding taking it. Young men and women are more likely to take the sorts of risks that would require emergency contraception than older clients (Pearson *et al.*, 1995), but are less likely to request it. This may be for a number of reasons, from lack of knowledge of its availability and awareness of its use, to concern over confidentiality and fear of a hostile reception. This indicates the need to inform clients about emergency contraception – they may never need the information themselves but may inform a friend. Men should not be forgotten when educating clients about emergency contraception; increasingly they are taking an interest and responsibility for contraception which should be encouraged. Often receptionists are forgotten in our zeal to educate, yet it is important that they are aware of the need for these clients to obtain immediate appointments. It is also important that they are aware of other clinics where emergency contraception is available, especially outside normal working hours, as they are most likely to receive telephone requests for this information. Giving emergency contraception can not only save a great deal of anguish over an unwanted pregnancy and abortion, but is also much more cost-effective and has less risk to the health of the woman.

ANSWERS TO SELF-ASSESSMENT QUESTIONS

1   *A woman with a regular cycle of 4/25 days attends requesting emergency contraception. It is 100 hours since the first episode of unprotected sexual intercourse, and she is now on day 20 of her cycle. Can you give her emergency contraception?*

Unfortunately, since she is more than five days from the earliest calculation of ovulation, an IUD cannot be fitted; she would ovulate between days 9 and 13. Because it is now 100 hours since her earliest episode of unprotected sexual intercourse she could have Ulipristal acetate, which is licensed for 120 hours, or the Levonorgestrel method, but the latter option would be unlicensed and the issue of limited data on efficacy over 96 hours would need to be discussed with her. You should advise her to return in three weeks' time for a pregnancy test if she has not had a normal menstrual period within that time. You should discuss future contraception and she could quick start on the POP or COC and use extra precautions depending on the type of hormonal emergency contraception given, or she could either use condoms or abstain from sexual intercourse and commence alternative contraception with her next period.

2   *What are the indications for emergency contraception?*

The indications for emergency contraception are as follows:

■   Unprotected sexual intercourse (e.g. condom break or misuse, diaphragm fitted incorrectly, no contraception used, missed pills, late injectable).
■   Rape and sexual assault.
■   Recent use of drugs with a teratogenic effect where unprotected sexual intercourse has taken place (e.g. cytotoxic drugs, live vaccines such as yellow fever).

14

FEMALE STERILIZATION

- Introduction and history
- Hysteroscopic sterilization
- Counselling a couple for female sterilization
- Procedure
- Post-female sterilization
- Reversal of female sterilization
- Sexuality and anxieties

INTRODUCTION AND HISTORY

Female sterilization is the only permanent method of female contraception. It was first mentioned by Hippocrates, but it was not until 1834 that Von Blundell fully described this method. At this time it was an extremely dangerous procedure involving abdominal surgery and hospitalization for long periods. In 1944 Drs Decker and Cherry reported on the successful outcomes of their culdoscopy procedure, which involved reaching the fallopian tubes through the vagina rather than through the abdomen. It was not until 1961 that laparoscopic sterilization was first described by Uchida.

Today, female sterilization is performed abdominally by either a mini-laparotomy or by laparoscopic sterilization. It can be performed as a day-care procedure either under a general or local anaesthetic.

Explanation of the method

Female sterilization involves excising or blocking the fallopian tubes which carry the ovum from the ovary to the uterus. This prevents the ovum from being fertilized by sperm in the fallopian tube.

Efficacy

Female sterilization is a highly effective form of contraception with a lifetime failure rate of one in 200 woman years. The effectiveness varies depending which method is used: diathermy and Filshie clips are considered the most effective. A retrospective study of the Filshie clip showed the failure rate to be between 2 and 3 per 1000 sterilization operations (Kovacs and Krins, 2002; RCOG, 2004).

Disadvantages

- Involves a surgical procedure and anaesthetic.
- Not easily reversed.

Advantages

- High efficacy.
- Permanent.
- Effective immediately.

Delay the procedure

- Post-partum under six weeks.
- Current venous thromboembolism using anti-coagulants.
- Major surgery.
- Immobility.
- Current ischaemic heart disease.
- Cervical, ovarian and endometrial cancer.
- Current PID or sexually transmitted infection.
- Current gall-bladder disease.

Caution required

- Request for sterilization at young age (e.g. under 25).
- Cerebrovascular accident.
- Obesity may be contra-indication for a laparoscopic procedure.
- Hypertension.
- Epilepsy.
- Depressive disorders.
- Valvular and congenital heart disease.

Range of method

Female sterilization involves excising or blocking the fallopian tubes by:

1 Applying a Hulka-Clemens or Filshie clip – this flattens and occludes the fallopian tube.
2 Drawing up a section of the fallopian tube and applying a Falope ring to the fallopian tube.
3 Excising and ligating the fallopian tube.
4 Sealing the fallopian tubes by intrafallopian implants.

Some of these methods are shown in Fig. 14.1.

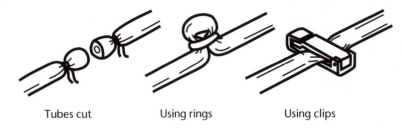

| Tubes cut | Using rings | Using clips |

Figure 14.1 Female sterilization techniques: tying the ends after the tubes have been cut; Falope ring; Filshie clip. (Adapted from FPA, 'Your guide to male and female sterilisation', November 2012, p. 9)

HYSTEROSCOPIC STERILIZATION

Using a hysteroscope, a guide wire places a flexible micro-insert into each fallopian tube; the micro-insert causes scar tissue to form, occluding the fallopian tube. This process can take three months to take effect, so alternative contraception is advised for the three months following the procedure. The procedure is performed under local anaesthetic by a specially trained doctor and takes 10 minutes. Occlusion of the fallopian tubes should be confirmed by ultrasound or X-ray (some women may need a hysterosalpingogram) before this method can be relied upon to prevent conception (NICE, 2009). Essure is a small titanium metal coil that can be fitted this way and is available in the UK.

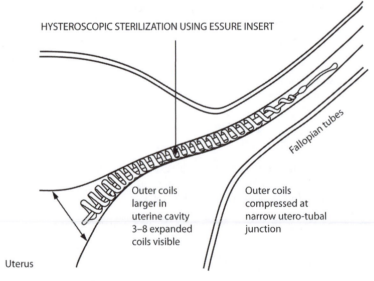

HYSTEROSCOPIC STERILIZATION USING ESSURE INSERT

Fallopian tubes

Outer coils larger in uterine cavity 3–8 expanded coils visible

Outer coils compressed at narrow utero-tubal junction

Uterus

Figure 14.2 Essure technique

- If there is a method failure then there is a higher risk of ectopic pregnancy.
- Feelings of grief and loss.

COUNSELLING A COUPLE FOR FEMALE STERILIZATION

Counselling a couple is extremely important for this procedure as it should be considered a permanent method. Careful counselling will also reduce post-operative regret and grief over the loss of fertility which some women experience.

During counselling with the couple you should discuss how they would feel if something happened to their children. How would they feel if something happened to their present partner – would they want children with a new partner? Are they both certain they do not want any more children? There are no set answers to these questions, but they are areas that need to be considered which can be difficult to discuss. It is important to give an unbiased view when discussing sterilization. You may hold personal views yourself about this method but these should not influence the couple in their decision. It is useful to meet the couple together, rather than the woman on her own, as the decision affects both parties and you may get different views and opinions about the decision. However, you may wish to complete the medical history with the woman on her own, as there may be details of her personal medical history that her partner is unaware of (e.g. previous abortion).

You should complete a full medical history of your client with special attention to gynaecological history. If, for example, she suffers from menorrhagia or dysmenorrhoea then this will continue following sterilization. In this situation it may be more appropriate for her to have the Levonorgestrel intrauterine system or undergo a hysterectomy, which would treat these symptoms. In the past, women often complained that a sterilization caused menorrhagia and dysmenorrhoea; this was more likely due to the fact that once they stopped the combined pill, which had reduced these symptoms, they returned to their true cycle following sterilization. Research (Rulin et al., 1993) undertaken to investigate the long-term effect of female sterilization on menses and pelvis pain showed no long-term difference between sterilized and non-sterilized women.

Women should be advised to continue with their present method of contraception until after the procedure, so that there is no chance of them being pregnant that cycle. If a woman uses an IUD as her method she should be advised to use condoms for the menstrual cycle prior to the procedure, to ensure that no sperm are present in the fallopian tubes, which could fertilize an ovum that is released shortly after surgery, resulting in an ectopic pregnancy.

You should discuss with your clients the efficacy and side effects of sterilization. Sterilization is a very effective form of contraception, but if it fails there is a higher risk of an ectopic pregnancy. You should discuss the difficulties of reversing this procedure so that a couple will understand fully the decision they are making. Sterilization should not be performed at a termination of pregnancy or following childbirth, as the failure rate is higher due to increased vascularity of the tissues involved, and there may also be regret of the decision made at this emotional time.

PROCEDURE

Female sterilization is usually performed under general or local anaesthetic and the most common procedure is laparoscopic sterilization. This is where a small incision is made at the umbilicus and the abdomen is filled with carbon dioxide gas. The operating table is tilted backwards, which ensures that all the other organs move away from the uterus. Using the laparoscope the fallopian tubes are located, and either ligated or clips applied. This procedure may be performed as a day case and, depending on home circumstances, it may be possible for the woman to go home that day.

If a woman has had previous gynaecological surgery or is obese it may not be possible to perform a laparoscopic sterilization. In this situation a mini-laparotomy may be indicated. This procedure involves a larger abdominal incision and usually requires hospitalization of four to five days. After the sterilization most surgeons perform a dilatation and curettage (D&C) to ensure that there is no risk of pregnancy following sexual intercourse prior to the procedure.

POST-FEMALE STERILIZATION

Following the procedure women may complain of cramp-like period pain for a few days as well as shoulder pain. This occurs as a result of using carbon dioxide gas and the application of the clips.

Women should be advised to seek medical attention immediately if they experience any signs of pregnancy or miss a menstrual period. This should be investigated to exclude an intrauterine or extrauterine pregnancy.

Women who experience regret over their decision and signs of grief and loss should be offered post-operative counselling, although counselling prior to the operation should reduce this problem.

REVERSAL OF FEMALE STERILIZATION

Female sterilization should be considered irreversible. Successful reversal will depend on the type of procedure used when the woman was initially sterilized, her age and the skill of the surgeon performing the reversal. The success rate in achieving pregnancy following reversal can be between 50 and 90 per cent, depending on the original method used. Following reversal a woman is at a higher risk of ectopic pregnancy, with 3 to 5 per cent of pregnancies being ectopic (Belfield, 1997).

The methods of sterilization which are most easily reversed are the use of Hulka or Filshie clips, as these flatten the fallopian tubes which can be re-inflated. Cautery and diathermy are the hardest to reverse, and are used less often these days because of the dangers of damaging other organs. The Falope ring can cause a portion of the fallopian tube to necrose, making reversal more difficult.

SELF-ASSESSMENT QUESTIONS

Answers and discussion at the end of the chapter.

1 Which women do you think are most suitable for female sterilization?
2 In what way is age relevant to a request for female sterilization?

SEXUALITY AND ANXIETIES

Women who have a sterilization often feel liberated – they no longer have the anxiety of pregnancy. Often a pregnancy scare precipitates a request for sterilization. This new-found freedom from anxiety enables many women to explore their own sexuality, and allows them to enjoy sexual intercourse in a way they have been unable to do before.

ANSWERS TO SELF-ASSESSMENT QUESTIONS

1   *Which women do you think are most suitable for female sterilization?*

Women who are most suitable for sterilization have completed their families and are in stable relationships. They have considered their future and thought carefully about all the options available to them.

2   *In what way is age relevant to a request for female sterilization?*

If a woman is under the age of 30 a request for sterilization needs to be treated with caution. There will be concern that a woman may change her mind and want to have more children, especially if something happens in her current relationship.

   Women who are older, in their forties, may have only a few fertile years left. It may be more appropriate for these women to choose a method with a high efficacy like Depoprovera, the IUS or an IUD like the T 380A range. Often women have not considered these methods.

15

PRECONCEPTUAL CARE

- Introduction
- Preconceptual care for men
- Preconceptual care for women
- Genetic counselling
- Socio-economic influences
- Sexuality and anxieties

INTRODUCTION

Family planning involves preconceptual counselling – many women do not think about becoming pregnant before it's too late. It is important to discuss this subject with women prior to conceiving to reduce the incidence of problems in pregnancy.

PRECONCEPTUAL CARE FOR MEN

Men wishing to conceive should follow certain guidelines.

Alcohol

Alcohol can damage a man's sperm, making it harder to conceive. Men are recommended to keep consumption low during this period.

Drugs

Illegal drugs can cause problems in conceiving. This is a good time to try and stop through counselling and support.

Smoking

Smoking can affect a man's sperm. This is a good time to stop smoking, as there is an increased risk of cot death if a parent smokes.

Sexually transmitted infections

Screening for sexually transmitted infections should be offered; this should include HIV and syphilis serology, chlamydia and gonorrhoea.

PRECONCEPTUAL CARE FOR WOMEN

Women planning to become pregnant should be advised to follow certain guidelines.

Diet

Women should be encouraged to eat a healthy diet low in fat and high in fibre. If they are overweight they should try to reduce their weight well ahead of conceiving, preferably at least three months beforehand, so that they do not have depleted stores of vitamins and minerals. Women who are underweight may have difficulty conceiving; they should be advised to eat three meals a day, with snacks in between.

Certain foods should be avoided in pregnancy. These include liver because of its high level of vitamin A, and foods made with uncooked eggs like mayonnaise and undercooked meat because of the risk of salmonella. Cheeses made with unpasteurized milk and mould ripened cheeses should be avoided (e.g. brie, camembert), as they may carry the bacteria Listeria which can lead to miscarriage and stillbirth, and serious illness in the unborn baby. Other foods which should be avoided include pâté and cooked chilled chicken, as these also carry the risk of these infections.

Alcohol

Alcohol should be reduced to no more than eight units a week and no more than two units a day in pregnancy.

Supplements

The Department of Health recommend that women take 400mg of folic acid prior to conceiving and until they are 12 weeks pregnant to prevent neural tube defects (Department of Health, 1992a).

Toxoplasmosis

This is a parasitic infection which can seriously affect the unborn foetus, causing brain damage and blindness. It is a flu-like illness which is contracted through raw meat, cat faeces, sheep and goat milk. Women should be advised to avoid handling cat litter trays, wash their hands when handling animals and wear gloves when gardening.

Smoking

Smoking should be avoided during pregnancy. It is a good idea to try and give up prior to pregnancy. Women who smoke in pregnancy are more likely to have a low birth weight baby which is associated with increased mortality and morbidity in the perinatal period and later in infancy (House of Commons Health Committee, 1990–1991).

Rubella

It is vital that women are routinely screened for rubella immunity prior to conceiving. If women are susceptible to rubella they should be immunized and avoid pregnancy for one month (BNF, 2012). If a woman is susceptible to rubella and contracts the disease during the first eight to ten weeks of pregnancy this can result in congenital rubella syndrome resulting in damage of 90 per cent of infants. Foetal abnormalities include learning disabilities, cataract, deafness, cardiac abnormalities, intrauterine growth retardation, and inflammatory lesion of the brain, lung, liver and bone marrow.

Sickle cell disease and thalassaemia

Women and men who are potential carriers of sickle cell disease and thalassaemia should be routinely screened. Those at risk of sickle cell disease are people of African, West Indian and occasionally of Asian origin, while those at risk of thalassaemia are of Mediterranean origin, particularly from Greece, Turkey and Cyprus, and also people from Pakistan and India. Screening and genetic counselling can reduce the incidence of these diseases.

Sexually transmitted infections and cervical cytology

Women should be encouraged to sort out any health problems they may have before becoming pregnant. Women should make sure that they have had a recent cervical smear and have regular dental check-ups. If there is any likelihood of a sexually transmitted disease being present then full screening should be performed and treatment given. For example, bacterial vaginosis, chlamydia, gonorrhoea and trichomoniasis are all associated with premature labour from premature rupture of membranes and as a result low birth weight, so screening can reduce problems in pregnancy.

Drugs and medication

Illegal drugs are harmful to the foetus. Women taking illegal drugs should try to obtain help and counselling prior to conceiving. Legally prescribed drugs should be taken with caution. Doctors and dentists should be advised by women that they are planning to get pregnant. If medication is taken that can be bought over the counter, women should check with the pharmacist that this safe to take at this time.

GENETIC COUNSELLING

Genetic counselling is offered to couples with a personal or family history of an inherited medical condition (e.g. cystic fibrosis, Down's syndrome). This gives couples the opportunity to make an informed decision following discussion about the facts of the condition concerned and risks involved. Genetic counselling involves discussion about the genetic abnormality and appropriate screening. A full history of the couple involved is taken and a family tree developed which will include the medical history of all family members. From this information the couple will be given an estimation of the risk to future pregnancies of the disorder occurring, and continued counselling and support will be offered so that they are enabled to come to a decision over future pregnancies.

SOCIO-ECONOMIC INFLUENCES

Many women become pregnant without seeking advice over health beforehand, while only a small minority of women actively seek help and advice in planning a pregnancy. As a result it is necessary for health care professionals to approach the subject of pregnancy with women at an appropriate opportunity. This will not only enable women to make adjustments in their diet and have preconceptual screening, but it also gives them time to consider the implications of a pregnancy in their life. This is particularly important for women who do not speak English as their first language, as they may have reduced access to literature in their own language. It is often unknown if a women is illiterate, which emphasizes the need to discuss issues verbally and how unreliable it is to expect men and women to read literature provided in waiting rooms.

Often the implications of a pregnancy are not considered until it is too late. In today's financial climate many couples have debts either to credit cards or in the form of negative equity with their mortgage, or perhaps they are unable to sell a property and are living in a property that is now too small for their family. Many men and women no longer believe that their employment is secure; they may not have a permanent contract with their employer or may have a short-term contract, which may cause them anxiety. It may be that by becoming pregnant money will be severely restricted, or employment will be at risk; not all employers are sympathetic to pregnancy. Although there is never a perfect time to become pregnant, a couple may be able to make some provisions for a pregnancy if they give time to consider the implications for them now, or they may decide to accept financial hardship or other problems following discussion with each other. By discussing these issues beforehand and negotiating their future, a couple are less likely to have problems within their relationship once the baby is born.

A pregnancy can cement a relationship, making it closer and stronger, but it can also be the final straw to an unsatisfactory one. Sometimes women mistakenly believe that a pregnancy will solve current relationship problems; usually this is the reverse. Occasionally there are situations when women have been so desperate to have children, because they see their time running out, that they have failed to look at their long-standing relationship with neglected psychosexual problems, which now have to be approached to achieve a pregnancy.

Today many women are the 'bread-winners' in families or their salary is a major part of the family income. This has put restrictions on the number of children couples choose to have. Women now delay pregnancy until they are older and their career is secure, but this causes many dilemmas as to when the best time for a pregnancy will be. There is of course no 'best time' for a pregnancy and this needs to be explored with clients. It may be that the couple have already left it too late and now have infertility problems, which can cause anger and distress within the relationship.

Women who are already single parents may be in this situation because of a pregnancy at a young age, a broken relationship, or where women have actively chosen to become pregnant as a single parent. Being a single parent is extremely hard, not only for the mother but also for the child involved. Today men and women live further away from their families so there is no close-knit family network to help with the upbringing of the child, so it all falls on one person.

When counselling men and women about preconceptual issues your personal views and attitudes should be hidden, so that a couple are able to reach their own decision. This can be very difficult, as couples will often ask whether you have children or what you would do in the given situation. It is important that their decision is their own, as however hard this may be they will be able to accept this more easily in the future if it is their own decision.

SEXUALITY AND ANXIETIES

Today many women delay pregnancy until they are in their thirties or forties and often fail to think about the implications of this decision. Because contraception is so effective, it has helped to delay the decision of pregnancy, creating a dilemma as women now have to actively stop contraception to become pregnant. Women may find it harder to become pregnant as they become older and this can increase their feelings of regret and guilt. Sometimes women find that they have left pregnancy too late and this can cause a great deal of anguish and heartache. With careful counselling these feelings may be able to be explored.

16

PREGNANCY: WANTED AND UNWANTED

- Introduction
- Negative pregnancy test
- Positive pregnancy test
- Symptoms of pregnancy
- Signs of pregnancy
- Pregnancy counselling
- Contraception following abortion
- Methods of abortion
- Complications of abortion
- Sexuality and anxieties

INTRODUCTION

Pregnancy is an area of great concern for women who attend for contraception and family planning advice. Women may consult concerned that they are unable to become pregnant; this may be connected to guilt over previous genito-urinary infections or terminations of pregnancy, or anxiety about using a method of contraception for a prolonged period like the combined oral contraceptive. Other women may consult unaware that they are at risk of pregnancy and this topic may need to be approached. Some women may already be aware that they are pregnant and require confirmation; they may also have made a decision about the future of this pregnancy. Other women may need time to consider their decision and discuss this with their partner.

If there is any suspicion that a woman may be pregnant, a pregnancy test should be performed to confirm this. Sometimes a woman can be so adamant that she is not pregnant that when a pregnancy test disproves this, she can find it hard to believe the test results. A pregnancy test should be performed one week after a missed period. It is useful to take a history which should include menstrual cycle length, episodes of unprotected sexual intercourse and contraception, along with any symptoms of pregnancy. Often a woman will tell you openly how she feels about a pregnancy, but if she does not discuss her feelings it is helpful to approach this subject prior to performing the test, as this will help you when you have to give her the results.

ACTIVITY

What abortion facilities are available locally? Why not see if you can visit so that you can ensure you are giving your clients up-to-date information?

NEGATIVE PREGNANCY TEST

If a pregnancy test is negative this may be because the test has been performed too early, or because the specimen is too dilute or too old, giving a false negative result. A false negative result may also be due to an ectopic pregnancy or a miscarriage, which will require further investigation if suspected. Details of menstrual cycle, contraception and any episodes of unprotected sexual intercourse should be ascertained. Any complaints of abdominal pain will necessitate further examination through pelvic ultrasound to exclude an ectopic pregnancy or miscarriage.

POSITIVE PREGNANCY TEST

If a pregnancy test is positive and a woman wishes to continue with the pregnancy she should self-refer to her general practitioner. However, sometimes women are unprepared for a positive result and may need time to discuss this with their partner. An appointment should be made at a convenient time, preferably with you, in the near future. It is useful to work out the gestation of the pregnancy, as this will give you an idea of when to see your client for a follow-up appointment. You should discuss the options available to her so that she can think about these and discuss them with her partner. Some women already have a suspicion that they are pregnant and have thought about their options already, basing a decision on their feelings.

It is important to allow a woman time to express her feelings. Many women will ask what you would do in this situation. It is important not to influence a client over her decision and to give non-judgemental counselling. A decision over an unwanted pregnancy is probably one of the hardest dilemmas a woman has to face, yet in the long term it will be easier if she has been allowed to make this decision herself; an empathetic approach will help her to do this.

SYMPTOMS OF PREGNANCY

Women may complain of the following symptoms of pregnancy:

- Nausea and vomiting.
- Increased micturition.
- Amenorrhoea.
- Breast changes.
- Skin changes.

SIGNS OF PREGNANCY

Certain signs help to confirm pregnancy:

- Positive pregnancy test.
- Enlarged uterus.
- Foetal heart sounds can be heard at 10 weeks by sonicaid ultrasonic equipment.
- Foetal movements felt.
- Foetal parts felt.
- Ultrasound may be used to diagnose pregnancy at six weeks.
- X-ray can show foetal skeletons at 14 to 16 weeks but should be avoided, as irradiation can damage the developing foetus.

PREGNANCY COUNSELLING

If a woman feels that she does not want to continue with her pregnancy she has two main options: she can have the baby adopted or have the pregnancy terminated with an abortion. These days it is rare for women to choose to have their baby adopted and most women will opt for an abortion. In 2011, 189,931 abortions were performed in England and Wales (National Statistics, 2012), and 47 per cent of women will choose a medical abortion over a surgical abortion. Ninety-six per cent of abortions were funded by the NHS, so providing and encouraging effective contraceptive use will not only prevent a woman from going through an emotional procedure but also saves the NHS money. The Royal College of Obstetricians and Gynaecologists (RCOG, 2011) has produced clinical guidelines for induced abortion, and these recommend ideally that:

- All women are offered an assessment appointment within five working days of referral.
- All women undergo an abortion within five working days of the decision to proceed and this should be no later than ten days.

Women can choose to have an abortion privately or through the National Health Service (NHS). If they wish to have an abortion via the NHS they may need to attend their local family planning clinic or GP for a referral to be made locally. If they choose to have a private abortion this should be at a clinic approved by the Department of Health for this procedure.

It is useful to give women a brief outline about the choices of abortion available. It is safer for a woman and less traumatic to have an abortion before 12 weeks. If a woman chooses to have a private abortion, an early abortion before 12 weeks will cost less and can be performed as a day case. Women often mistakenly believe that they will have the abortion at the initial consultation. They should be warned that this appointment usually involves the completing of a medical history. Usually a pregnancy test is repeated and an ultrasound examination will be performed to confirm gestation and exclude ectopic pregnancy. Women will receive pre-abortion counselling at this appointment and a date for the abortion procedure will be organized. If at any stage a woman wishes to change her mind about her decision she may do so at any point. As this is such a difficult decision this does sometimes happen, and it is important that she is aware that she has this opportunity.

ACTIVITY

Do you know where women can be referred locally for private and NHS abortions?
Do you know how much a private abortion would cost in your area?

An abortion may be carried out under the 1967 Abortion Act if two registered medical doctors find that it is necessary on one or more counts prior to 24 weeks' gestation. These are that if the pregnancy were to continue it would involve risk to the life of the woman, or would cause injury to her physical or mental health, or would cause injury to existing children's physical or mental health. Finally, if there is a substantial risk of the child being born with physical or mental abnormalities. An amendment to this Act in 1991 reduced the upper limit from 28 to 24 weeks' gestation, but in special circumstances this limit does not apply. These circumstances are when the life of the woman is at risk or there is a possibility of permanent injury, or when there is serious foetal handicap.

You should encourage your client to return after the procedure for a follow-up appointment so that she can discuss how she feels and any problems can be approached. It is a good idea to encourage your client to undergo a screen for sexually transmitted infections such as chlamydia and gonorrhoea, HIV and syphilis; this should be performed along with the provision of contraception. Women may not have considered contraception following the procedure, so it is useful to discuss this and, if possible, provide it so that it can be commenced immediately after the abortion; this will help reduce any anxiety afterwards. Women often say 'never again' so they are only too happy to discuss contraception, and may choose a different method, as they may have a loss of confidence if they have had a method failure.

CONTRACEPTION FOLLOWING ABORTION

The diaphragm and cervical cap should be refitted following an abortion in case a new size is required, while the IUS and IUD may be inserted immediately following a first trimester abortion. Following a termination of pregnancy Nexplanon may be inserted immediately; if inserted later, additional contraception will be required for seven days. Depoprovera may be given within the first seven days with no extra precautions required, while POP and COC should be commenced the same day or the next day with no additional precautions required following a first trimester abortion.

METHODS OF ABORTION

The main methods of abortion are as follows:

1 Surgical abortion, which can be carried out by:

- Vacuum aspiration.
- Dilatation and curettage (D&C).
- Dilatation and evacuation (D&E).

2 Medical abortion.

Surgical abortion

Vacuum aspiration

This is where the cervix is dilated under general anaesthetic and the contents of the uterus emptied by suction. This is the most widely used method and is carried out before 12 weeks' gestation, usually as a day case.

Dilatation and curettage (D&C)

The cervix is dilated and a curette is introduced into the uterus and the contents removed. This is usually carried out under general anaesthetic.

Dilatation and evacuation (D&E)

Again, this is performed under general anaesthetic. The cervix is dilated and the contents of the uterus emptied. Vacuum aspiration is then performed. This method is usually performed in second trimester abortions and may be undertaken up to 20 weeks, although it is preferable to do this before 16 weeks to reduce the risks of a late abortion.

Medical abortion

A medical abortion may be carried out if a pregnancy is less than or equal to 63 days' gestation, which is confirmed by ultrasound scan. It involves, following counselling, the administration of oral Mifepristone 200mg tablets on day 1 with an observation period of two hours. If the woman vomits within this period she will have to be referred for a surgical abortion. Some women experience vaginal bleeding and period-like abdominal cramps. Abdominal pain should not be treated with non-steroidal anti-inflammatory drugs (NSAIDS) (e.g. aspirin, ibuprofen, mefenamic acid), but other analgesics may be given. Contact telephone numbers are given. If heavy bleeding is experienced or there is severe pain, clients may need to be admitted earlier.

This is followed 24 to 48 hours later if under 63 days' gestation with Misoprostol 800 micrograms given by the vagina, buccal or sublingual route or, if under 49 days of gestation, 200mg of Mifepristone followed 24 to 48 hours later with 400 micrograms of Misoprostol orally. She is observed for six hours in order to monitor blood pressure and any problems which may be experienced. Vaginal bleeding usually begins within two hours after administration and may continue for 12 days, gradually lessening. Women will experience abdominal pain, and the abortion should occur within the six-hour period.

A follow-up and ultrasound should be offered if successful abortion has not been confirmed to exclude continuing pregnancy.

Contra-indications

- Pregnancy exceeding 64 days' gestation.
- Suspected ectopic pregnancy.

- Allergy to mifepristone.
- Chronic adrenal failure.
- Long-term corticosteriod therapy.
- Haemorrhagic disorders.
- Anti-coagulant treatment.
- Smokers aged over 35.

Relative contra-indications

- Asthmatics and chronic obstructive airways disease.
- Cardiovascular disease.
- Renal or hepatic disease.
- Women with prosthetic heart valves.
- Pregnancies of 56 to 63 days' gestation.

Side effects

Drug-related side effects:

- Nausea.
- Vomiting.
- Diarrhoea.
- Faintness.
- Hot flushes.

Side effects related to treatment:

- Infection.
- Abdominal pain.
- Bleeding.

COMPLICATIONS OF ABORTION

- Failure to end pregnancy (risk fewer than 1 in 100).
- Uterine rupture (risk 1 in 1000).
- Retained products of conception and surgical intervention (risk less than 5 per cent).

There have been concerns that abortion is associated with breast cancer, and research (Goldbeck-Wood, 1994) has shown an association between abortion and breast cancer; however, almost all the studies have been retrospective (Birth Control Trust, 1994). The Royal College of Obstetricians and Gynaecologist has found no evidence to support an increased risk of breast cancer with induced abortion (RCOG, 2011). There is no increased risk of placenta praevia, infertility or ectopic pregnancy following abortion; however, there is a small increased risk of pre-term birth.

SEXUALITY AND ANXIETIES

An unwanted pregnancy brings many anxieties to women. Even if the decision to have an abortion seems to be right for them, there are inevitably regrets. Women may experience the various stages of grief over their decision: denial, anger, depression and acceptance. How they cope with this loss will depend on the counselling and support they receive. Many women subconsciously remember the date of the abortion and the estimated date of delivery. Often they expect to be chastised for their mistake by professionals, and caution should be taken over women who wish to have a medical abortion or surgical abortion with local anaesthetic who feel that in some way they should suffer for their present situation.

Women who have recurrent abortions may be desperately trying to seek help. There may be relationship problems and/or feelings of loss of self-worth underlying their cry for attention. Given time and counselling these feelings may be able to be approached and explored.

Sometimes women use unplanned pregnancy and abortion to test their relationship, which can cause problems within it. However, it can also bring a couple closer together. Women may become pregnant shortly after this episode, but this time continues with the pregnancy.

Following abortion, women may choose to change their method of contraception, as they may experience a loss of faith in it. A review (Hudson and Hawkins, 1995) of contraceptive practices before and after an abortion showed that following abortion women changed their method to one with a higher efficacy, generally a hormonal method. Many women following an abortion experience a great deal of anxiety about becoming pregnant again, and may consult more with pregnancy scares. Often clients hold misconceptions about abortion; they may believe that their future fertility is affected and this can cause a great deal of guilt.

BIBLIOGRAPHY

Albert, A.E., Warner, D.L., Hatcher, R.A., Trussell, J. and Bennett, C. (1995) Condom use among female commercial sex workers in Nevada's legal brothels. *American Journal of Public Health* **85**: 1514–1520.

Allen, M.E. (ed.) (1991) *Good Clinical Practice in Europe. Investigator's Handbook*, pp. 19–35. Romford: Rostrum Publications.

American Health Consultants (2000) Femcap in Germany, seeking U.S. approval. Contraceptive Technology Update, pp. 35–36.

Andersson, K., Mattsson, L-M., Rybo, G. and Stadberg, E. (1992) Intrauterine release of levonorgestrel – a new way of adding progestogen in hormone replacement therapy. *Obstetrics and Gynaecology* **79**: 963–967.

Andersson, K., Odlind, V. and Rybo, G. (1994) Levonorgestrel-releasing and copper releasing (Nova T) IUDs during five years of use: A randomised comparative trial. *Contraception* **49**: 56–72.

Aubeny, E., Colau, J-C. and Nandeuil, A. (2000) Local spermicidal contraception: A comparative study of the acceptability and safety of a new pharmaceutical formulation of benzalkonium chloride, the vaginal capsule, with a reference formulation, the pessary. *The European Journal of Contraception and Reproductive Health Care* **5**: 61–67.

Bagwell, M.A., Coker, A.L., Thompson, S.J., Baker, E.R. and Addy, C.L. (1995) Primary infertility and oral contraceptive steroid use. *Fertility and Sterility* **63**: 1161–1166.

Bekele, B. and Fantahun, M. (2012) The Standard days method: An addition to the arsenal of family planning method choice in Ethiopia. *Journal of Family Planning Reproductive Healthcare* **38**: 157–166.

Belfield, T. (1997) *FPA Contraceptive Handbook*, 2nd edn. London: Family Planning Association (FPA).

Benner, P. (1994) *From Novice to Expert*. Menlo Park, CA: Addison-Wesley.

Birth Control Trust (1994) Briefing: Possible association between abortion and breast cancer. Letter.

Birth Control Trust (1997) *Abortion Provision in Britain: How Services are Provided and How They Could be Improved*. London: Birth Control Trust.

Bjarnadottir, R.I., Gottfredsdottir, H., Sigurddardottir, K., Geirsson, R.T. and Dieben, T.O.M. (2001) Comparative study of the effects of a progestogen only pill containing desogestrel and an intrauterine device in lactating women. *British Journal of Obstetrics and Gynaecology* **108**: 1174–1180.

Black, T. (2003) Comparison of Marie Stopes scalpel and electrocautery no-scalpel vasectomy techniques. *The Journal of Family Planning and Reproductive Sexual Health Care* **29**: 32–34.

Blain, S., Oloto, E., Meyrick, I. and Bromham, D. (1996) Skin reactions following Norplant insertion and removal – possible causative factors. *The British Journal of Family Planning* 21: 130–132.

BMA, GMSC, HEA, Brook Advisory Centres, FPA and RCGP (1993) Joint guidance note: *Confidentiality and People Under 16.* British Medical Association, General Medical Science Committee, Health Education Authority, Brook Advisory Centres, Family Planning Association and Royal College of General Practitioners.

Bonn, D. (1996) What prospects for hormonal contraceptives for men? *The Lancet* 347: 316.

Bonnar, J., Flynn, A., Freundl, G., Kirkman, R., Royston, R. and Snowden, R. (1999) Personal hormone monitoring for contraception. *The British Journal of Family Planning* 24: 128–134.

Bontis, J., Vavilis, D., Theodoridis, T. and Sidropoulou, A. (1994) Copper intrauterine contraceptive device and pregnancy rate. *Advances in Contraception* 10: 205–211.

Bounds, W. (1994) Contraceptive efficacy of the diaphragm and cervical caps used in conjunction with a spermicide – a fresh look at the evidence. *The British Journal of Family Planning* 20: 84–87.

Bounds, W. and Guillebaud, J. (2002) Observational series on women using the contraceptive Mirena concurrently with anti-epileptic and other enzyme-inducing drugs. *The Journal of Family Planning and Reproductive Health Care* 28: 78–80.

Bounds, W., Kubba, A., Tayob, Y., Mills, A. and Guillebaud, J. (1986) Clinical trial of a spermicide-free, custom-fitted, valved cervical cap (Contracap). *British Journal of Family Planning* 11: 125–131.

Bounds, W., Guillebaud, J. and Newman, G.B. (1992a) Female condom (Femidom). A clinical study of its use-effectiveness and patient acceptability. *The British Journal of Family Planning* 18: 36–41.

Bounds, W., Hutt, S., Kubba, A., Cooper, K., Guillebaud, J. and Newman, G.B. (1992b) Randomised comparative study in 217 women of three disposable plastic IUCD thread retrievers. *British Journal of Obstetrics and Gynaecology* 99: 915–919.

Bounds, W., Robinson, G., Kubba, A. and Guillebaud, J. (1993) Clinical experience with a levonorgestrel-releasing intrauterine contraceptive device (LNG-IUD) as a contraceptive and in the treatment of menorrhagia. *The British Journal of Family Planning* 19: 193–194.

Bounds, W., Guillebaud, J., Dominik, R. and Dalberth, B. (1995) The diaphragm with and without spermicide. A randomised, comparative efficacy trial. *The Journal of Reproductive Medicine* 40: 764–774.

Bounds, W., Molloy, S. and Guillebaud, J. (2002) Pilot study of short-term acceptability and breakage and slippage rates for the loose-fitting polyurethane male condom eZ.on bi-directional: A randomized cross-over trial. *The European Journal of Contraception and Reproductive Health Care* 7: 71–78.

Brahams, D. (1995) Medicine and the law: Warning about natural reversal of vasectomy. *The Lancet* 345: 444.

British National Formulary (BNF) (2012) *British National Formulary.* London: BMJ Group and Pharmaceutical Press.

Bromham, D.R. (1996) Contraceptive implants. *British Medical Journal* 312: 1555–1556.

Canter, A.K. and Goldthorpe, S.B. (1995) Vasectomy – patient satisfaction in general practice: A follow up study. *The British Journal of Family Planning* **21**: 58–60.

Cardy, G.C. (1995) Outcome of pregnancies after failed hormonal postcoital contraception – an interim report. *The British Journal of Family Planning* **21**: 112–115.

Chantler, E. (1992) Vaginal spermicides: Some current concerns. *British Journal of Family Planning* **17**: 118–119.

Chilvers, C. (1994) Breast cancer and depot-medroxyprogesterone acetate: A review. *Contraception* **49**: 211–222.

Clubb, E. and Knight, J. (1996) *Fertility*. Newton Abbot: David & Charles.

Collaborative Group on Hormonal Factors in Breast Cancer (1996a) Breast cancer and hormonal contraceptives: Collaborative reanalysis of individual data on 53 297 women with breast cancer and 100 239 woman without breast cancer from 54 epidemiological studies. *The Lancet* **347**: 1713–1727.

Collaborative Group on Hormonal Factors in Breast Cancer (1996b) Breast cancer and hormonal contraceptives. *Contraception* **54**: 3 (supplement).

Collaborative Study Group on the Desogestrel Progestogen-only pill (1998) A double blind study comparing the contraceptive efficacy, acceptability and safety of two progestogen only pills containing desogestrel 75 micrograms/day or Levonorgestrel 30 micrograms/day. *The European Journal of Contraception and Reproductive Health Care* **3**: 169–178.

Committee on Safety of Medicines (CSM) (2002) Current problems in pharmacovigilance. *Medicines Control Agency* 28.

Conor, S. and Kingman, S. (1988) *The Search for the Virus. The Discovery of AIDS and the Quest for a Cure*. London: Penguin Books.

Coutinho, E.M., De Souza, J.C., Athayde, C., Barbosa, I.C., Alvarez, F., Brache, V., Zhi-Ping, G., Emuveyan, E.E., Adeyemi, O., Devoto, L., Shaabam, M.M., Salem, H.T., Affandi, B., Mateo de Accosta, O., Mati, J. and Ladipo, O.A. (1996) Multi centre clinical trial on the efficacy and acceptability of a single contraceptive implant of Normegestrol Acetate, Uniplant. *Contraception* **53**: 121–125.

Cox, M. (2002) Clinical performance of the Nova T380 intrauterine device in routine use by the UK Family Planning and Reproductive Health Research Network: 5 year report. *The Journal of Family Planning and Reproductive Health Care* **28**: 69–72.

Crosier, A. (1996) Women's knowledge and awareness of emergency contraception. *The British Journal of Family Planning* **22**: 87–90.

CSAC (1993a) Long term progestogen only contraception (injection and oral) and effect on oestrogen. *British Journal of Family Planning* **18**: 134–135.

CSAC (1993b) Retention of IUDs after the menopause. *British Journal of Family Planning* **18**: 134–135.

Cundy, T., Evans, M., Roberts, H., Wattie, D., Ames, R. and Reid, I.R. (1991) Bone density in women receiving depot medroxyprogesterone acetate for contraception. *British Medical Journal* **303**: 13–16.

Cundy, T., Cornish, J., Evans, M.C., Roberts, H. and Reid, I.R. (1994) Recovery of bone density in women who stop using medroxyprogesterone acetate. *British Medical Journal* **308**: 247–248.

Cushman, L.F., Davidson, A.R., Kalmuss, D., Heartwell, S. and Rulin, M. (1996) Beliefs about Norplant Implants among low income urban women. *Contraception* **53**: 285–291.

Dalton, K. (1983) *Once a Month*. Glasgow: Fontana.

Daly, M. and Mansour, D. (2002) *Yasmin: A New Option in Contraception. Purchaser Profile*. Guildford: Schering Health Care and A&M Publishing.

Darney, P., Klaisle, C.M., Tanner, S. and Alvarado, A.M. (1990) Sustained release contraceptives. *Current Problems in Obstetrics, Gynaecology and Fertility* **13**: 99–100.

Davidson, J.A.H. (1992) Warming lignocaine to reduce pain associated with injection. *British Medical Journal* **305**: 617–618.

de Jong, F.H. (1987) Inhibin – its nature, site of production and function. In Clarke, J.R. (ed.) *Oxford Review of Reproductive Biology*, Vol. 9. Oxford: Oxford University Press.

Dennis, J. and Hampton, N. (2002) IUDs: Which device? *The Journal of Family Planning and Reproductive Health Care of the Royal College of Obstetricians and Gynaecologists* **28**: 61–68.

Dennis, J., Webb, A. and Kishen, M. (2001) Expulsions following 1000 GyneFix insertions. *Journal of Family Planning Reproductive Health Care* **27**: 135–138.

Department of Health (1992a) *Folic Acid and Neural Tube Defects: Guidelines on Prevention*. London: Department of Health (Letter).

Department of Health (1992b) *Immunisation against Infectious Disease*. London: HMSO.

Department of Health (1995) The response for doctors to the Committee on Safety of Medicines letter. FPA and Faculty of Family Planning and Reproductive Health Care of the Royal College of Obstetricians and Gynaecologists.

Department of Health (1999) *Teenage Pregnancy*. London: Department of Health.

Department of Health (2002) *The National Strategy for Sexual Health and HIV: Department of Health*. London: Department of Health.

Diaz, J., Faundes, A., Olmos, P. and Diaz, M. (1996) Bleeding complaints during the first year of Norplant implants use and their impact on removal rate. *Contraception* **53**: 91–95.

Drug and Therapeutics Bulletin (1996a) Topiramate – add on drug for partial seizures. *Drug and Therapeutics Bulletin* **34**: 62–64.

Drug and Therapeutics Bulletin (1996b) Hormone replacement therapy. *Drug and Therapeutics Bulletin* **34**: 81–84.

Drug and Therapeutics Bulletin (2002) Copper IUDs, infection and infertility. *Drug and Therapeutics Bulletin* **40**: 67–69.

Durex (1993) *History of the Condom*. London: Durex Information Service.

Durex (1994) *The Durex Report 1994: A Summary of Consumer Research into Contraception*. London: Durex Information Service.

Durex network (2010) *The Face of Global Sex 2010 – They Won't Know Unless We Tell Them*. London: SSL International PLC.

The Economist (1995) On the needles hounding of a safe contraceptive. Science and technology. *The Economist*, 2 September, pp. 113–114.

Editorial (1996) Pill scares and public responsibility. *The Lancet* **347**: 1707.

Edwards, J.E. and Moore, A. (1999) Implanon. A review of clinical studies. *The British Journal of Family Planning* **24**: 3–16.

European Medicine Agency (EMA) (2013) Start of review of combined hormonal contraceptives containing chloramadinone, desogestrel, dienogest, drospirenone, etonogestrel, gestodene, normestrol, norelgestromin or norgestimate. European Medicines Agency.

Faculty of Family Planning and Reproductive Health Care (FFPRHC) (2000)

FFPRHC Guidance April 2000 Emergency Contraception: Recommendations for clinical practice. *Journal of Family Planning and Reproductive Health Care*.

Faculty of Family Planning and Reproductive Health Care (FFPRHC) (2003) FFPRHC Guidance Emergency Contraception. Faculty of Family Planning and Reproductive Health Care Clinical Effectiveness Unit. *Journal of Family Planning and Reproductive Health Care* **29**: 9–16.

Faculty of Family Planning and Reproductive Health Care (FFPRHC) (2007) FFPRHC Clinical Guidance Male and Female Condoms. Faculty of Family Planning and Reproductive Health Care Clinical Effectiveness Unit.

Faculty of Family Planning and Reproductive Health Care of the Royal College of Obstetricians and Gynaecologists (1996) Statement on hormonal contraceptives and breast cancer, Thursday 20 June 1996 (Letter).

Faculty of Sexual and Reproductive Healthcare (2007) Clinical Guidance: Intrauterine contraception. Faculty of Sexual and Reproductive Healthcare.

Faculty of Sexual and Reproductive Healthcare (2008a) Recommendations from the CEU: Antibiotic prophylaxis for intrauterine contraceptive use in women at risk of bacterial endocarditis. Faculty of Sexual and Reproductive Healthcare.

Faculty of Sexual and Reproductive Healthcare (2008b) Progestogen only injectable contraception. Clinical Effective Unit, Faculty of Sexual and Reproductive Healthcare.

Faculty of Sexual and Reproductive Healthcare (2008c) Progestogen only implants. Clinical Effective Unit, Faculty of Sexual and Reproductive Healthcare.

Faculty of Sexual and Reproductive Healthcare (2008d) Progestogen only pills. Clinical Effective Unit, Faculty of Sexual and Reproductive Healthcare.

Faculty of Sexual and Reproductive Healthcare (2009a) (revised 2010) UK medical eligibility criteria for contraceptive use. Faculty of Sexual and Reproductive Healthcare.

Faculty of Sexual and Reproductive Healthcare (2009b) Management of unscheduled bleeding in women using hormonal contraception. Faculty of Sexual and Reproductive Healthcare.

Faculty of Sexual and Reproductive Healthcare (2009c) Combined vaginal ring. NuvaRing. Contraception Clinical Effectiveness Unit, Faculty of Sexual and Reproductive Healthcare.

Faculty of Sexual and Reproductive Healthcare (2010a) Quick starting contraception. Clinical Effectiveness Unit, Faculty of Sexual and Reproductive Healthcare.

Faculty of Sexual and Reproductive Healthcare (2010b) Service standards for resuscitation. Faculty of Sexual and Reproductive Healthcare.

Faculty of Sexual and Reproductive Healthcare (2010c) Contraception for women aged over 40 years. Clinical Effectiveness Unit, Faculty of Sexual and Reproductive Healthcare.

Faculty of Sexual and Reproductive Healthcare (2011a) Combined hormonal contraception. Clinical Effectiveness Unit, Faculty of Sexual and Reproductive Healthcare.

Faculty of Sexual and Reproductive Healthcare (2011b) (updated January 2012) Drug interactions with hormonal contraception, Clinical Effectiveness Unit. Faculty of Sexual and Reproductive Healthcare.

Faculty of Sexual and Reproductive Healthcare (2012a) Emergency contraception. Clinical Effectiveness Unit, Faculty of Sexual and Reproductive Healthcare.

Faculty of Sexual and Reproductive Healthcare (2012b) Barrier methods for contraception and STI prevention. Clinical Effectiveness Unit, Faculty of Sexual and Reproductive Healthcare.

Faculty of Sexual and Reproductive Healthcare (2012c) Risk of venous thrombosis in users of non oral contraceptives. Statement from the Faculty of Sexual and Reproductive Healthcare.

Faculty of Sexual and Reproductive Healthcare (2013) Use of Ulipristal Acetate (ellaOne®) in breastfeeding women. Update from the Clinical Effectiveness Unit, Faculty of Sexual and Reproductive Healthcare.

Farley, T.M.M., Rosenberg, M.J., Rowe, P.J., Chen, J-H. and Meirik, O. (1992) Intrauterine devices and pelvic inflammatory disease: An international perspective. *The Lancet* **339**: 785–788.

Farr, G. and Amatya, R. (1994) Contraception and efficacy of the copper T 380A and copper T 200 intrauterine devices: Results from a comparative clinical trial in six developing countries. *Contraception* **49**: 231–243.

Farr, G., Amatya, R., Doh, A., Ekwempu, C.C., Toppozada, M. and Ruminjo, J. (1996) An evaluation of the copper-T 380A IUD's safety and efficacy at three African centers. *Contraception* **53**: 293–298.

Flynn, A. (1996) Natural family planning. *The British Journal of Family Planning* **21**: 146–148.

Ford, N. and Mathie, E. (1993) The acceptability and experience of the female condom, Femidom among family planning clinic attenders. *The British Journal of Family Planning* **19**: 187–192.

Fowler, P. (1996) Subdermal implants – still a viable long-term contraceptive option? *The British Journal of Family Planning* **22**: 31–33.

FPA (1993) *Vasectomy and Prostrate Cancer*. London: Family Planning Association.

FPA (1995) FPA Fact File 3B: *Contraception: Some Factors Affecting Research and Development*. London: Family Planning Association.

Frezieres, R.G., Walsh, T.L., Nelson, A.L., Clark, V.A. and Coulson, A.H. (1999) Evaluation of the efficacy of a polyurethane condom: Results from a randomized, controlled clinical trial. *Family Planning Perspectives* **31**: 81–87.

Gbolade, B.A. (2002) Depoprovera and bone density. *The Journal of Family Planning and Reproductive Health Care* **28**: 7–11.

Gillmer, M.D., Walling, M.R. and Povey, S.J. (1996) The effect on serum lipids and lipoproteins of three combined oral contraceptives containing norgestimate, gestodene and desogestrel. *The British Journal of Family Planning* **22**: 67–71.

Giovannucci, E., Ascherio, A., Rimm, E., Colditz, G.A., Stampfer, M.J. and Wilett, W.C. (1993a) A prospective cohort study of vasectomy and prostate cancer in US men. *Journal of the American Medical Association* **269**: 873–877.

Giovannucci, E., Tosteson, T.D., Speizer, F.E., Ascherio, A., Vessey, M.P. and Colditz, G.A. (1993b) A retrospective cohort study of vasectomy and prostate cancer in US men. *Journal of the America Medical Association* **269**: 878–882.

Glasier, A.F., Cameron, S.T., Fine, P.M., Logan, S.J.S., Casale, W., Van Horn, J., Laszlo, S., Blithe, D.L., Scherres, B., Mathe, H., Jaspart, A., Ulmann, A. and Gainer, E. (2010) Ulipristal acetate versus levonorgestrel for emergency contraception: A randomised non inferiority trial and meta analysis. *The Lancet* **375**: 555–562.

Goldbeck-Wood, S. (1994) Researchers claim abortion increases risk of breast cancer. *British Medical Journal* **313**: 962.

Gooder, P. (1996) Knowledge of emergency contraception amongst men and women in the general population and women seeking an abortion. *The British Journal of Family Planning* 22: 81–84.

Grady, W.R., Klepinger, D.H., Billy, J.O.G. and Tanfer, K. (1993) Condom characteristics: The perceptions and preferences of men in the United States. *Family Planning Perspective* 25: 67–73.

Guillebaud, J. (1997) *Contraception Today*, 3rd edn. London: Martin Dunitz.

Guillebaud, J. (1999) *Contraception: Your Questions Answered*, 3rd edn. Edinburgh: Churchill Livingstone.

Guillebaud, J. and Bounds, W. (1983) Control of pain associated with intrauterine device insertion using mefenamic acid. *Research and Clinical Forums* 5: 69–74.

Ho, P.C. and Kwan, M.S.W. (1993) A prospective randomised comparison of levonorgestrel with the Yuzpe regimen in post-coital contraception. *Human Reproduction* 8: 389–392.

Hollingworth, B. and Guillebaud, J. (1994) The levonorgestrel intrauterine device. *The Diplomate* 1: 247–251.

House of Commons Health Committee (1990–1991) *Maternity Services: Preconception*. London: HMSO (Fourth report, Vol. 1).

Howards, S.S. and Peterson, H.B. (1993) Vasectomy and prostate cancer. Chance, bias or a causal relationship. *Journal of the American Medical Association* 269: 913–914.

Hudson, G. and Hawkins, R. (1995) Contraception practices of women attending for termination of pregnancy – a study from South Australia. *The British Journal of Family Planning* 21: 61–64.

Hughes, H. and Myers, P. (1996) Women's knowledge and preference about emergency contraception: A survey from a rural general practice. *The British Journal of Family Planning* 22: 77–78.

Ikomi, A. and Pepra, E.F. (2002) Efficacy of the Levonorgestrel intrauterine system in treating menorrhagia: Actualities and ambiguities. *The Journal of Family Planning and Reproduction Health Care* 28: 99–100.

Indian Council of Medical Research Task Force on Natural Family Planning (1996) Field trial of Billings ovulation method of natural family planning. *Contraception* 53: 69–74.

International Family Planning Perspectives (1992) Invasive cervical cancer risk no greater for DMPA users than for nonusers. *International Family Planning Perspectives* 18: 156–157.

Janssen-Cilag International N.V. (2003) Summary of product characteristics. Janssen-Cilag International N.V. Belgium.

Jick, H., Jick, S.S., Gurewich, V., Myers, M.W. and Vasilakis, C. (1995) Risk of idiopathic cardiovascular death and nonfatal venous thromboembolism in women using oral contraceptives with differing progestagen components. *The Lancet* 346: 1589–1592.

Kovacs, G.T. and Krins, A.J. (2002) Female sterilization with Filshie clips: What is the risk failure? A retrospective survey of 30,000 applications. *The Journal of Family Planning and Reproductive Health Care* 28: 34–35.

Leiras (1995) Mirena levonorgestrel 20 micrograms/24 hours. Product monograph. Finland: Leiras.

Lewis, M.A., Spitzer, W.O., Heinemann, L.A.J., Macrae, K.D., Bruppacher, R. and Thorogood, M. (1996) Third generation oral contraceptives and risk of myocardial infarction: An international case control study. *British Medical Journal* 312: 88–90.

Lidegaard, O., Hougaard Nielson, L., Wessel Skovlund, C. and Lokkegaard, E. (2012) Venous thrombosis in users of non oral hormonal contraception: Follow-up study, Denmark 2001–10. *British Medical Journal* 344: e2990.

Luukkainen, T. (1993) The levonorgestrel releasing IUD. *British Journal of Family Planning* 19: 221–224.

McCann, M.F. and Potter, L.S. (1994) Progestin-only oral contraception: A comprehensive review. *Contraception* 50: S3–S195.

McEwan, H. (1990) The menopause. In Pfeffer, N. and Quick, A. (eds) *Promoting Women's Health*. London: King Edward's Hospital Fund for London.

Machin, S.J., Mackie, I.J. and Guillebaud, J. (1995) Factor V Leiden mutation, venous thromboembolism and combined oral contraceptive usage. *British Journal of Family Planning* 21: 13–14.

Mackie, I.J., Piegsa, K., Furs, S.A., Johnson, J., Bounds, W., Machin, S.J. and Guillebaud, J. (2001) Protein S levels are lower in women receiving desogestrel-containing combined oral contraceptives (COCs) than in women receiving levonorgestrel-containing COCs at steady state and on cross-over. *British Journal of Haematology* 113: 898–904.

Marchbanks, P.A., McDonald, J.A., Wilson, H.G., Folger, S.G., Mandel, M.G. and Daling, J.R. (2002) Oral contraceptives and the risk of breast cancer. *New England Journal of Medicine* 346: 2025–2032.

Mascarenhas, L., Newton, P. and Newton, J. (1994) First clinical experience with contraceptive implants in the U.K. *British Journal of Family Planning* 20: 60 (Letter).

Masters, T., Everett, S., May, M. and Guillebaud, J. (2002) Outcomes at 1 year for the first 200 patients fitted with GyneFix at Margaret Pyke Centre. *The European Journal of Contraception and Reproduction Health Care* 7: 65–70.

Mauk, C., Glover, L.H., Miller, E., Allen, S., Archer, D.F., Blumenthal, P., Rosenzweig, B.A., Dominik, R., Sturgen, K., Cooper, J., Fingerhut, F., Peacock, L. and Gabelnick, H.L. (1996) Lea's Shield: A study of the safety and efficacy of a new vaginal barrier contraceptive used with and without spermicide. *Contraception* 53: 329–333.

Mishell, D.R. (ed.) (1994) Papers presented at a World Health Organisation meeting on Once-a-month combined injectable contraception – Part I. *Contraception* 49: 291–420.

National Institutes of Health (1993) Final statement – March 2, 1993. Vasectomy and Prostate Cancer Conference USA. Family Health International. Bethseda, MD: National Institute of Child Health and Human Development.

National Statistics (2012) *Abortion Statistics in England and Wales: 2011*. London: Department of Health.

NICE (2009) *Hysteroscopic Sterilisation by Tubal Annulation and Placement of Intrafallopian Implants. Interventional Procedure Guidance 315. N1995*. London: National Institute for Health and Clinical Excellence.

Niruthisard, S., Roddy, R. and Chutivongse, S. (1991) The effects of frequent Nonoxynol-9 use on the vaginal and cervical mucosa. *Sexually Transmitted Diseases* 18: 176–179.

Nursing and Midwifery Council (NMC) (2008) *The Code*. London: Nursing and Midwifery Council.

Organon (1998) *Summary of Product Characteristics*. Cambridge: Organon Laboratories.

Organon (2002) *Implanon Implant for Subdermal Use.* Cambridge: Organon Laboratories.

Parkes, A.S. (1976) *Patterns of Sexuality and Reproduction.* Oxford: Oxford University Press.

Pearson, V.A.H., Owen, M.R., Phillips, D.R., Pereira Gray, D.J. and Marshall, M.N. (1995) Pregnant teenagers' knowledge and use of emergency contraception. *British Medical Journal* 310: 1644.

Pharmacovigilance Working Party (PhVWP) (2011) Ethinylestradiol and Drospirenone containing oral contraceptives – Risk of venous thromboembolism. European Medicine Agency.

Pisake, L. (1994) Depot-medroxyprogesterone acetate (DMPA) and cancer of the endometrium and ovary. *Contraception* 49: 203–209.

The Population Council (1990) *Norplant Levonorgestrel Implants: A Summary of Scientific Data.* New York: The Population Council.

Prabakar, I. and Webb, A. (2012) Emergency contraception. *British Medical Journal* 344: 1492.

Psychoyos, A., Creatsas, G., Hassan, E., Georgoulias, V. and Gravanis, A. (1993) Spermicidal antiviral properties of cholic acid: Contraceptive efficacy of a new vaginal sponge (Protectaid) containing sodium cholate. *Human Reproduction* 8: 866–869.

Raudaskoski, T.H., Lahti, E.I., Kauppila, A.J., Apajasarkkinen, M.A. and Laatikainen, T.J. (1995) Transdermal estrogen with a levonorgestrel-releasing intrauterine device for climacteric complaints: Clinical and endometrial responses. *American Journal of Obstetrics and Gynaecology* 172: 114–119.

Rice, C.F., Killick, S.R., Dieben, T. and Coelingh Bennink, H. (1999) A comparison of the inhibition of ovulation achieved by desogestrel 75 micrograms and Levonorgestrel 30 micrograms. *Human Reproduction* 14: 982–985.

Robinson, G.E. (1994) Low-dose combined oral contraceptives. *British Journal of Obstetrics and Gynaecology* 101: 1036–1041.

Robinson, G.E., Bounds, W., Kubba, A., Judith, A. and Guillebaud, J. (1989) Functional ovarian cysts associated with the levonorgestrel releasing device. *British Journal of Family Planning* 14: 131–132.

Roddy, R.E., Cordero, M., Cordero, C. and Fortney, J.A. (1993) A dosing study of nonoxynol-9 and genital irritation. *International Journal of STD & AIDS* 4: 165–170.

Roussel Laboratories Ltd (1994) *Norplant Product Review.* London: Haymarket Medical Imprint.

Royal College of Obstetricians and Gynaecologists (2004) *Male and Female Sterilisation.* Evidence-based Clinical Guideline No. 4. London: RCOG Press.

Royal College of Obstetricians and Gynaecologists (2011) *The Care of Women Requesting Induced Abortion.* Evidence-based Clinical Guideline No. 7. London: RCOG Press.

Rulin, M.C., Davidson, A.R., Philliber, S.G., Graves, W.L. and Cushman, L.F. (1993) Long-term effect of tubal sterilization on menstrual indices and pelvic pain. *Obstetrics and Gynaecology* 82: 118–121.

Ruminjo, J.K., Amatya, R.N., Dunson, T.R., Kruegers, S.L. and Chi, I.C. (1996) Norplant implants acceptability and user satisfaction among women in two African countries. *Contraception* 53: 101–107.

Ryan, P.J., Singh, S.P. and Guillebaud, J. (2002) Depot medroxyprogesterone and bone mineral density. *The Journal of Family Planning and Reproductive Health Care* 28: 12–15.

Ryder, B. and Campbell, H. (1995) Natural family planning in the 1990s. *The Lancet* 346: 233–234.

Saracco, A., Musicco, M., Nicolosi, A., Angarano, G., Arici, C., Gavazzeni, G., Costigliola, P., Gafa, S., Gervasoni, C., Luzzati, R., Piccinino, F., Puppo, F., Turbessi, G., Vigevani, G.M., Visco, G., Zerboni, R. and Lazzarin, A. (1993) Man-to-woman sexual transmission of HIV: Longitudinal study of 343 steady partners of infected men. *Journal of Acquired Immune Deficiency Syndromes* 6: 497–502.

Short, R.A. (1994) Contraceptives of the future in the light of HIV infection. *Australian New Zealand Obstetric Gynaecology* 34: 330–332.

Sibai, B.A., Odlind, V., Meador, M.L., Shangold, G.A., Fisher, A.C. and Creasy, G.W. (2002) A comparative and pooled analysis of the safety and tolerability of the contraceptive patch (Ortho Evra). *Fertility And Sterility* 77: S20–26.

Simms, M. (1993) Teenage pregnancy – give girls a motive for avoiding it. *British Medical Journal* 306: 1749–1750 (Letter).

Sinai, I., Lundgren, R.I. and Gribble, J.N. (2012) Continued use of the Standard Days Method. *Journal of Family Planning Reproductive Healthcare* 38: 150–156.

Sivin, I. (1988) International experience with Norplant and Norplant 2 contraceptives. *Studies in Family Planning* 19: 81–94.

Sivin, I. and Stern, J. (1994) Health during use of levonorgestrel 20 mg/d and the copper TCU 380Ag intrauterine contraceptive devices: A multicenter study. *Fertility and Sterility* 61: 70–77.

Smith, T. (1993) Influence of socio economic factors on attaining targets for reducing teenage pregnancies. *British Medical Journal* 306: 1232–1235.

Sparrow, M.J. and Lavill, K. (1994) Breakage and slippage of condoms in family planning clients. *Contraception* 50: 117–129.

Spitzer, W.O., Lewis, M.A., Heinemann, L.A.J., Thorogood, M. and Macrae, K.D. (1996) Third generation oral contraceptives and risk of venous thromboembolic disorders: An international case-control study. *British Medical Journal* 312: 83–88.

Steinke, E. (1994) Knowledge and attitudes of older adults about sexuality in ageing: A comparison of two studies. *Journal of Advanced Nursing* 19: 477–485.

Suhonen, S., Lahteenmaki, P., Haukkamaa, M., Rutanen, E.-M. and Holstrom, T. (1996) Endometrial response to hormone replacement therapy as assessed by expression of insulin-like growth factor-binding protein 1 in the endometrium. *Fertility and Sterility* 65: 776–782.

Task Force on Postovulatory Methods of Fertility Regulation (1998) Randomised controlled trial of Levonorgestrel versus the Yuzpe regimen of combined oral contraceptives for emergency contraception. *The Lancet* 352: 428–433.

Trimmer, E. (1978) *Basic Sexual Medicine*. London: Heinemann Medical.

Trussell, J. and Stewart, F. (1992) The effectiveness of postcoital hormonal contraception. *Family Planning Perspectives* 24: 262–264.

Trussell, J., Sturgen, K., Stickler, J. and Dominik, R. (1994) Comparative contraceptive efficacy of the female condom and other barrier methods. *Family Planning Perspectives* 26: 66–72.

UK Family Planning Research Network (1993) Mishaps occurring during condom use, and the subsequent use of post-coital contraception. *British Journal of Family Planning* 19: 218–220.

Veos UK (2001) Oves the new contraceptive cap. *Draft Medical Information Handbook*. London: Veos UK.

Vessey, M.P. (1988) Urinary tract infection and the diaphragm. *British Journal of Family Planning* **13**: 41–43.

Vessey, M.P., Lawless, M., Yeates, D. and McPherson, K. (1985) Progestogen-only oral contraception. Findings in a large prospective study with special reference to effectiveness. *British Journal of Family Planning* **10**: 121–126.

Vessey, M.P., Villard-Mackintosh, L. and Yeates, D. (1990) Effectiveness of progestogen only oral contraceptives. *British Journal of Family Planning* **16**: 79 (Letter).

Vessey, M.P., Yeates, D. and Flynn, S. (2010) Factors affecting mortality in a large cohort study with special reference to oral contraceptive use. *Contraception* **82**: 221–229.

Vincenzi, I. de (1994) A longitudinal study of human immunodeficiency virus transmission by heterosexual partners. *New England Journal of Medicine* **331**: 341–346.

Von Hertzen, H., Piaggio, G., Ding, J., Chen, J., Song, S., Bartfai, G., Ng, E., Gemzell-Danielsson, K., Oyunbileg, A., Shangchun, W., Cheng, W., Ludicke, F., Bretnar-Darovec, A., Kirkman, R., Mittal, S., Rhomassuridze, A., Apter, D. and Peregoudov, A. (2002) Low dose mifepristone and two regimens of Levonorgestrel for emergency contraception: A WHO multicentre randomized trial. *The Lancet* **360**: 1803–1810.

West, R.R. (1992) Vasectomy and testicular cancer – no association on current evidence. *British Medical Journal* **304**: 729–730.

WHO (1981) *Research on the Menopause*. World Health Organization Technical Report No. 670. Geneva: WHO.

WHO (1991) World Health Organization Collaborative Study of Neoplasia and Steroid Contraceptives. Breast cancer and depot-medroxyprogesterone acetate: a multinational study. *The Lancet* **338**: 833–838.

WHO (1992) World Health Organization Collaborative Study of Neoplasia and Steroid Contraceptives (1992) Depot medroxyprogesterone acetate (DMPA) and risk of invasive squamous cell cervical cancer. *Contraception* **45**: 299–312.

WHO (1995) World Health Organization Collaborative Study of Cardiovascular Disease and Steroid Hormone Contraception. Venous thromboembolic disease and combined oral contraceptives: Results of international multicentre case control study. *The Lancet* **346**: 1575–1581.

Wildemeersch, D., Van Kets, H., Vrijens, M., Van Trappen, Y., Temmerman, M., Batar, I., Barri, P., Martinez, F., Iglesias-Cortit, L. and Thiery, M. (1994) IUD tolerance in nulligravid and parous women: Optimal acceptance with the frameless CuFix implant (GyneFix). Long-term results with a new inserter. *British Journal of Family Planning* **20**: 2–5.

Wilson, E. (1993) Depoprovera: Underused and undervalued. *British Medical Journal* **18**: 101.

Wilson, E.W. and Rennie, P.I.C. (1976) *The Menstrual Cycle*. London: Lloyd-Luke.

Ziebland, S., Maxwell, K. and Greenhall, E. (1996) 'It's a mega dose of hormones, isn't it?' Why women may be reluctant to use emergency contraception. *British Journal of Family Planning* **22**: 84–86.

Zieman, M., Guillebaud, J., Weisberg, E., Shangold, G.A., Fisher, A.C. and Creasy, G.W. (2002) Contraception efficacy and cycle control with the Ortho Evra transdermal system: The analysis of pooled data. *Fertility and Sterility* **77**: S13–18.

INDEX